Inner Fire

Self-Care and Wellness for Winter

By
Ruby M. Waters

Inner Fire

Self-Care and Wellness for Winter

Table of Contents

Introduction

The chill in the air, the crispness of the morning frost, and the serene silence that winter brings offer us a unique opportunity to embark on a journey inward. While the world outside turns a little more introspective and slow, we too can embrace this season as a time for nurturing warmth and resilience within ourselves. Winter, despite its reputation for harshness, can be a season filled with possibilities of renewal and self-discovery. This book serves as a guide for those who seek to find balance and well-being amid the cold, darkness, and stillness.

For centuries, cultures worldwide have revered winter as a period of reflection and retreat. The trees shed their leaves, animals hibernate, and the landscape rests under a blanket of snow, silently preparing for the cycle of growth to resume in spring. Similarly, we can interpret this season as an invitation to pause, reflect, and embark on a voyage of self-care tailored to the unique challenges and gifts of winter.

Embracing winter might initially seem like a daunting task, especially when the colder months often conjure feelings of melancholy or fatigue. Yet, this is precisely why cultivating practices that welcome warmth and foster inner harmony is essential. By transforming how we relate to winter, we can shift from enduring the season to cherishing it as an integral part of our holistic well-being—and there are myriad ways to achieve this transformation.

As the days grow shorter, our natural inclination might be to retreat into our homes. Instead of viewing this as a limitation, we can view it as an opportunity—a chance to create a sanctuary conducive to comfort and introspection. Simple rituals, such as lighting a candle or indulging in a long bath, can become acts of transformation that restore our inner vitality. Understanding the enlightenment that can come from darkness is key to harnessing the true potential of this season.

Connecting with nature is another vital element for maintaining warmth in the winter months. Whether it's through a brisk walk in the crisp air or inviting the natural world indoors through plants and natural scents, nurturing this bond offers profound insights and peace. Even in winter, nature is very much alive, teaching invaluable lessons about adaptability and resilience.

Mindfulness and meditation further deepen our capacity to remain balanced and resilient. The quiet and introspective quality of winter provides an ideal backdrop for these practices. Taking moments to breathe deeply and acknowledge our presence in the now anchors us firmly in our inner warmth—even while the wind howls outside.

Winter is also a time to celebrate the joys of companionship and connection. Gathering with loved ones, sharing warm meals, and nurturing relationships play a significant role in fostering a sense of community and support. In a world where technology often isolates, genuine talks and shared laughter become even more precious.

The notion of self-care in winter isn't limited to the tangible; it also involves feeding the soul through creativity. Engaging in arts, music, and other forms of self-expression can be both invigorating and therapeutic. Art becomes a partner in our winter journey, helping articulate emotions and sparking joy.

Perhaps most crucially, this winter can be a season to explore personal growth and transformation. As leaves transform into spring blossoms, so too can the quiet strength cultivated in winter fuel our growth. This transformation isn't merely an annual cycle—it's a metaphor for continual personal development.

By intentionally embracing winter with a carefully cultivated practice of self-care and reflection, we open ourselves to a rich tapestry of experiences, strength, and serenity. This book offers a guide—a framework to draw upon as you cultivate your own journey and journey through the winter months.

Let this text be a beacon of inspiration and a call to action: to go forth into the winter, shedding the layers that no longer serve us while allowing our inner light to shine even the dimmest days.

Chapter 1:
Embracing Winter

As the world around us transforms with the hush of winter, there's a certain magic waiting to be discovered beneath its frosty surface. This time of year invites us to slow down and listen to the whisper of the cold wind as it carries wisdom and reflection. Winter's embrace is about finding solace in the quiet moments, those pockets of peace that offer a retreat from the clamour of everyday life. While the chill may bite, it's paired with an intrinsic beauty that unveils itself to anyone open to seeing the possibilities for growth and self-care. By welcoming winter with open arms, we allow ourselves to cultivate resilience, converting the often harsh solitude of the season into a powerful ally in our journey towards inner warmth and well-being. This harmonious dance with winter provides a unique opportunity to deepen our connection with ourselves, realigning our energy with the natural cycles of change and renewal.

Understanding the Season

Winter is often portrayed as a season of dormancy, a time when nature seems to pause, conserving its energy for the renewal of spring. But to truly understand winter, we need to look deeper, beneath the surface interlaced with frosted landscapes and bracing winds. It's a season brimming with profound lessons — it teaches the value of patience, the strength found in resilience, and the beauty in stillness.

The earth appears to be at rest, yet it's silently preparing for the burst of life that comes with the thawing of snow. In this way, winter offers an opportunity for reflection and renewal. Just as nature slows down, we too are encouraged to pace ourselves, finding balance and rejuvenating from within. It's a season that reminds us of the importance of self-care, urging us to slow down and listen to our inner voice.

Winter ushers in its own kind of beauty, distinct from the vibrant colours of spring or the warmth of summer. It bestows upon us scenes of breathtaking serenity — snow-covered landscapes that engage the senses in wholly different ways. The stark, bare trees stand as a testament to perseverance, echoing the silent resilience we possess within ourselves. In these moments of stillness, there's a space to cultivate inner warmth and well-being.

Yet, understanding winter is not merely about the outer world; it calls for a journey inwards. It's an invitation to connect deeply with our inner selves, finding warmth amid the cold. Just as nature adapts to the short days and longer nights, we can learn to embrace the quietude and solitude that winter encourages. These moments of introspection can become nurturing, offering insights into our own strength and capacity for growth.

Embracing winter also means acknowledging the challenges it brings — the colder temperatures, the shorter daylight hours, and the potential for feelings of isolation. But within these challenges lie opportunities to cultivate personal resilience. Using the season as a time to learn about balancing light and dark, warmth and cold, activity and rest, we discover ways to create harmony in our own lives.

One cannot truly understand the season without appreciating its natural cycles: the ebb and flow that mirrors our own lives. Winter is a time of rest and recharge. It's not about fighting against the cold and dark, but rather finding ways to navigate them with grace. Activities that invigorate the body and mind, from warming foods to nurturing relationships, become essential components of a well-rounded winter routine. By creating rhythms and practices that foster well-being, we can better harness the season's potential.

Moreover, winter's rhythm invites us to reassess our priorities and deepen our connection with what nourishes us. From the quiet moments with a steaming cup of herbal tea to the brisk outdoor walks that awaken our senses, there is a richness to winter waiting to be discovered. It encourages us to look at life's essentials from a fresh perspective, advocating for simplicity and presence.

Through an awareness of winter's offerings, we can tap into the wisdom it holds. It teaches us adaptation and acceptance, revealing that every season, every phase of life, holds its own treasures and opportunities. We learn the art of patience and resilience, appreciating the beauty in stillness and introspection.

Understanding winter is about embracing the calm it brings. It's about cultivating an inner sanctuary amidst the external chill, finding joy in small moments and cherishing the warmth of connection — both with others and oneself. As we align with the grace of this season, we find that winter, in all its silent splendour, teaches us to thrive.

In its essence, winter dares us to see beyond the chill and darkness, to find light and warmth within ourselves. It's a season that mirrors the potential within us, urging us to explore, reflect, and grow. As we navigate this time with openness and intention, we come to understand that winter isn't just a season to endure, but one to embrace and celebrate, for it holds the seeds of renewal that promise transformation come spring.

The Benefits of Winter's Quietude

Winter possesses a unique serenity that speaks to the soul. The world slows down as the days become shorter and temperatures drop. This seasonal pause isn't just a shift in weather; it's an invitation to embrace silence and stillness, offering gifts of reflection and self-awareness. Many of us might initially resist this profound quietude, perceiving it as isolation or inactivity. Yet, within this narrative of peace and calm lies an incredible opportunity for personal growth and rejuvenation.

During the colder months, nature itself retreats. Trees stand bare and dormant, yet beneath the surface, life persists and prepares for renewal. This seasonal hush mirrors our own inner landscapes. By aligning with winter's innate rhythm, we grant ourselves permission to slow down and enter a state of introspection. This quietude isn't about doing nothing—it's about doing less of what's unnecessary and more of what nourishes the spirit.

Winter's stillness can refresh the mind. With fewer distractions, we can focus inward, exploring facets of ourselves that often go unnoticed in busier times. Without the noise, we hear our own thoughts more clearly. Simple pleasures, like the crackle of a fire or the crunch of snow underfoot, become more pronounced, inviting us to appreciate the world in a different light. In embracing the quiet, we open ourselves to a deeper understanding of our needs and desires.

The seasonal quietude also allows for much-needed rest. Our modern lives are frequently characterised by unending activity and demands. Winter provides a natural counterbalance, a reminder to rest and recuperate. The physical and mental benefits of taking time to unwind are well-documented. When we slow down, we recover vital energies, preparing ourselves for the months ahead with renewed vigour and strength.

Moreover, winter offers space for creativity to blossom. When external stimuli are reduced, our minds start to expand inwardly. This is a time when many find themselves exploring creative pursuits—writing, art, music—that they might neglect in more bustling seasons. The quiet encourages us to express ourselves and delve into projects that require the patience and focus that only solitude can afford.

In addition to nurturing creativity, winter's quietude fosters deep connection. With less emphasis on external activities, relationships with family, friends, and oneself can be profoundly strengthened. Conversations take on a new depth when the world outside is hushed, offering moments to listen and be heard. Whether it's sharing a meal or engaging in heartfelt dialogue, these experiences root us in the fundamentals of human connection.

Winter's quietude is also a sanctuary for the spirit. Many spiritual traditions herald the colder months as a time for reflection and renewal. This quiet season offers a sacred pause, an opportunity to connect with spiritual practices that resonate on a deeply personal level. Whether through meditation, prayer, or simply being present, the serene silence of winter underscores a profound truth—peace is found within.

This reflective time allows us to cultivate gratitude. When stripped of the constant hum of daily life, we're better positioned to recognise the blessings we often overlook. The simplicity of winter invites a practice of appreciation, highlighting the beauty in starkness and the value of warmth both physical and emotional. It's a time to acknowledge the small joys and comforts that sustain us.

While the world quiets, we're given the chance for inner dialogue. We often find answers in the stillness that elude us in the din of daily life. These revelations are not always grand or life-altering, but they are genuine and aligned with who we are at our core. By embracing winter's hush, we enable profound discoveries about our values, ambitions, and the paths we wish to follow.

Embracing winter's quietude is not without its challenges. The dark, cold months can bring feelings of isolation, particularly if one isn't accustomed to being solitary. It's essential to balance our quiet reflection with social interactions and activities that bring joy. Yet, for those willing to lean into the stillness, this seasonal period offers some of the most rewarding opportunities for personal growth and transformation.

Ultimately, the silence of winter is a teacher. It reminds us of the cyclical nature of life and the importance of rest and renewal. As we integrate this seasonal rest into our lives, we might find ourselves more resilient against life's challenges, more attuned to our own rhythms, and more appreciative of the quiet beauty that surrounds us. In welcoming the gifts of winter's quietude, we set a foundation for the flourishing that follows in spring.

Chapter 2:
Nourishing Foods for Winter

As the chill of winter seeps into every corner, embracing the season with warmth begins on your plate. Winter foods, rich and hearty, are not just about feeding the body—they're about nurturing the soul. Imagine the comforting aroma of slow-cooked meals, their steam rising as they bring essence back into weary bones. The act of preparing nourishing foods becomes a ritual of self-care, where you thoughtfully select seasonal ingredients. Root vegetables, with their earthy depth, pair perfectly with soups and stews that envelop you like a snug blanket, while the zing of spices invigorates tired senses. This season, let your kitchen become a haven of warmth, crafting meals that bring balance and resilience amidst the stark beauty of winter. Embrace this culinary journey that sustains your inner fire and connects you with nature's cycles, fortifying you against the cold with every delightful bite.

Seasonal Ingredients

As winter takes its icy hold, the natural world offers us an array of ingredients that not only nourish the body but also provide warmth and comfort to the soul. Embracing these seasonal ingredients is not merely a culinary choice; it's a way of aligning ourselves with nature's rhythm, gaining strength from its abundance. The earth provides us with these treasures just when we need them the most, urging us to savour the tastes and textures that winter brings.

Root vegetables, often the unsung heroes of the winter produce aisle, take centre stage during the colder months. Carrots, parsnips, turnips, and beetroots, with their vibrant hues and earthy flavours, possess an innate ability to ground and nourish us. Their dense textures become a vehicle for comforting stews and hearty soups, melding together to create warmth in every spoonful. Indeed, the humble potato alongside sweet potatoes offers versatility, whether mashed, roasted, or blended into creamy potages.

Brassicas such as kale, cabbage, and Brussels sprouts also bloom under the winter skies. They thrive in the chill, bringing bitter, yet robust flavours which, when cooked, reveal a natural sweetness that pairs particularly well with warming spices like cumin and mustard seeds. These greens offer a bounty of nutrients, packed with vitamins and minerals that fortify our defences during the season. Experiencing the snap of fresh kale or the richness of slow-cooked cabbage is to engage with winter's bounty in its most healthful form.

Turning the page to fruits, winter is synonymous with citrus. Oranges, grapefruits, lemons, and limes enliven our senses with their refreshing tang and bright colours. These fruits don't just uplift our mood with their sunny disposition; they're also potent sources of vitamin C, essential for maintaining our immune systems. Enjoying a juicy orange or lemon-infused tea can be an act of self-care, adding zest to the often-grey winter days.

Apples and pears, usually associated with the harvest, remain relevant in the winter pantry. Stored properly, they provide a sweet counterpoint to savoury dishes or can be transformed into comforting desserts. Baked with spices or simmered into sauces, they remind us of the simple joys found in familiar flavours. These fruits serve as a gentle reminder of autumn's generosity, their resilience carrying us through the stark landscapes of winter.

Alongside fruits and vegetables, grains such as barley, oats, and quinoa are storehouses of nourishment. Their hearty nature makes them ideal companions for winter's chill, providing sustained energy and warmth. A steaming bowl of oatmeal for breakfast or a rustic barley risotto for dinner showcases the satisfying depth these grains bring to the winter table, often enriched further with nuts and dried fruits for added texture and taste.

Don't overlook the humble legumes either—beans, lentils, and chickpeas are indispensable during winter. They introduce a remarkable degree of versatility and substance to meals. Their protein-rich profiles are essential for maintaining energy levels, while their comforting, filling nature feels like a warm embrace. Lentil stews with spices or a chickpea curry can nourish the physical and emotional layers of our being.

Moreover, sourcing these ingredients locally and seasonally also breathes life into the community, supporting local farms and reducing our ecological footprint. Engaging with seasonal produce helps forge a deeper connection to the land and its cycles, encouraging mindfulness in our consumption. This practice is in itself a rhythm of nourishment, teaching us sustainability and gratitude for the earth's provisions.

Incorporating these seasonal ingredients into our winter menus isn't merely about flavour—it's an opportunity to fortify our bodies against the cold and nurture resilience. With each meal thoughtfully prepared, we imbue our days with the energy and vitality that only nature's seasonal gifts can provide. Through this intimate dance with the earth's cycles, we find warmth, balance, and an unshakeable well-being to carry us through winter's embrace.

Cooking Warm and Hearty Meals

As the chill of winter settles in, there's an innate desire to seek out warmth. It's not just about bundling up with more layers but finding ways to bring inner comfort and nourishment. One of the most fulfilling ways to achieve this is through the art of cooking. Warm, hearty meals not only satisfy our physical hunger but also nurture the soul, creating a sense of well-being and contentment. This ritual of making meals to share—either with loved ones or in solitude—has been a grounding practice for centuries.

Winter offers the perfect backdrop to delve into the creation of comforting dishes that celebrate the season's offerings. Root vegetables like carrots, potatoes, and turnips manage to capture the earth's warmth, while grains such as rice and barley provide hearty comfort. These ingredients aren't just meant to fill plates; they transform kitchens into spaces of warmth and creativity. Imagine the rustic simplicity of a stew simmering slowly on the stove, filling the air with its inviting aroma.

There's a meditative quality to preparing winter meals, a chance to be fully present in the act of creation. Chopping vegetables, stirring pots, seasoning to taste—each step is a mindful practice. This process allows us to connect to the food we're making, turning ingredients into a nourishing experience. Taking the time to cook not only feeds the body but establishes a rhythm that brings calm amidst the season's challenges.

The blend of spices is another aspect not to be overlooked. Ingredients like cinnamon, nutmeg, and cloves can transform a dish into a winter delight. They carry with them not just warmth but a host of beneficial properties that support our health during colder months. They add depth to dishes, inviting us to slow down and savour each bite. Spices engage our senses fully, evoking memories and emotions that further embed us into the season's embrace.

Casseroles, stews, and soups are quintessential winter comfort foods that reflect culinary traditions from around the world. These meals are characterised by their ability to be cooked at leisure, allowing flavours to meld over time. They are forgiving and adaptable, welcoming whatever ingredients you have at hand. Each dish becomes a blend of textures and flavours, a symphony of nourishment that can be as simple or as complex as your mood dictates.

Baking, too, finds its peak in winter months, as ovens hum with the promise of freshly baked bread and pastries. The act of baking is one of transformation—simple ingredients become magical through the process of mixing, kneading, rising, and baking. The resulting warmth from the oven spreads throughout the home, a comforting background to whatever winter throws your way. There's a profound satisfaction in breaking bread with others, an act that symbolises sharing, togetherness, and gratitude.

Winter meals aren't just about the food on the table; they're structured around moments of unity and reflection. Mealtimes become gatherings where people come together to share stories, laughter, and warmth. The dining table turns into a stage for connections, with each meal a chance to strengthen bonds and create cherished memories. It's a time to celebrate traditions and perhaps even craft new ones in the spirit of mindfulness and gratitude.

Yet, cooking in winter isn't solely about indulgence. It's a balance—a dance between nourishing comfort and mindful eating. Our bodies crave different nutrients in the colder months, often requiring a delicate balance of proteins, healthy fats, and complex carbohydrates. Each meal presents an opportunity to meet these needs actively, crafting plates that are not just hearty but healthful.

As you explore these culinary pursuits, allow yourself to be creative. Venture into trying new recipes or improvising with seasonal ingredients, guided by your taste and intuition. Winter is a canvas, a period to experiment with what nourishes both body and soul. Look to cookbooks for inspiration or experiment with family recipes handed down through the years. Each choice is a step towards creating warmth in your life.

Cooking warm and hearty meals becomes a journey, one that's shared across generations and cultures. It's a timeless practice, rooted in the rhythms of the earth and celebrated through the heart's strongest bonds. In the kitchen, with warmth radiating from the stove and aroma wafting through the air, we find a profound connection to winter itself. It's an invitation to embrace the season in all its forms—a passageway to inner warmth and resilience.

Chapter 3:
Creating a Cozy Home Environment

As winter's embrace closes in, creating a snug haven within your home becomes essential for nurturing your well-being and inner warmth. Crafting a cozy home environment isn't just about aesthetics; it's a beautiful interplay of comfort and tranquillity that fortifies your spirit against the cold outside. Drawing on the simple yet profound philosophy of hygge, seek out soft textiles, warm lighting, and inviting spaces that encourage relaxation and peace. Introduce aromatic scents that evoke memories of comfort, like cinnamon or vanilla, as they drift gently through the air, soothing the senses. Turning your home into a sanctuary means embracing a mindful approach to your surroundings, making space for both stillness and joy, while fostering an environment that supports your existing self-care practices. This gentle transformation lays the foundation for resilience, allowing you to greet each new day with quiet strength and positivity.

Hygge Essentials

As the frosty air settles in, embracing the Danish concept of hygge can be your key to cultivating warmth and contentment in your home. Pronounced "hoo-ga", it's not just about candles and blankets — it's a way of life that embodies comfort, solace, and camaraderie. At its core, hygge is about creating a sanctuary where you can escape the chill of winter, both outside and within your spirit.

Imagine stepping into a room softly aglow with the gentle flicker of candlelight. The sheer simplicity of a single candle can transform the atmosphere of a space, turning it into a warm embrace. Choosing candles made from eco-friendly materials such as soy or beeswax can add an environmentally mindful aspect to your hygge experience. Opt for scents like cinnamon or pine, which embody the essence of winter warmth.

Furniture arrangement can add another dimension to your cosy haven. Consider nooks filled with cushions and throws where you can curl up with a book or muse reflectively over a cup of tea. The tactile sensation of soft wool or the smooth surface of leather adds to the sensory experience, inviting you to touch, rest, and breathe. Don't shy away from mixing textures, as various fabrics juxtaposed together create visual and sensory richness.

The art of hygge also champions surrounding yourself with meaningful objects. Display mementos or items collected from nature, like twigs, stones, or seashells. These pieces can act as gentle reminders of personal journeys and cherished memories. Their presence not only enlivens the space but also connects you with the narrative of your life, a comforting balm during long, winter nights.

A harmonious colour palette in your home plays a significant role in fostering a hyggelig atmosphere. Neutral tones such as grey, beige, and pale blues simulate the calmness of snowy landscapes and promote relaxation. These subtle shades invite natural light in, maximising its warming effect even on the crispiest days. Pairing these hues with warm accents like terracotta or deep burgundy can add layers of warmth and depth.

No hygge environment is complete without the gentle hum of shared moments with loved ones. Whether it's a simple tea party or a board game night, it's the company that counts. Indeed, sharing is at the core of hygge — it encourages inclusion, laughter, and conversation free from haste and distraction. These gatherings foster a sense of belonging and build a warm tapestry of connections and joy.

Culinary delights also play their part in weaving hygge into everyday living. Winter is the ideal time to indulge in steaming bowls of soup, slow-cooked meals, and spiced pastries — dishes that nourish not just the body but the soul. The preparation and enjoyment of these meals can be a communal activity, further enriching the sense of togetherness and wellbeing.

Beyond tangible elements, hygge is about being mindful of the present moment. It's the contentment found in solitude and the invitation to reflect. Winter provides the perfect backdrop; the stillness outside mirrors the introspection within. A gentle meditative practice, like sitting quietly by the window and watching snowflakes dance in the wind, can bring profound peace.

Hygge nurtures gratitude, inviting you to appreciate the simple joys that surface throughout the cold months. It implores you to reflect on the year gone by and to envisage the path ahead. Perhaps it's a log fire's crackle, the rhythmic cadence of knitting needles, or the ambient tunes of a favourite playlist. Such elements enrich the hygge tapestry, encouraging a more profound connection with the present.

Lastly, the hygge mindset can extend beyond the confines of your home. Apply its principles to your daily life by wearing comforting clothing, practising gratitude, and prioritising moments of calm. Even the routine commute or a trip to the shops can be gezellig when approached with a hygge heart, transforming ordinary experiences into moments of joy.

As the snow dusts the landscape and the night draws in earlier, let the spirit of hygge envelop you. By embracing its essentials — warmth, togetherness, and simplicity — you forge an oasis of comfort that both welcomes you in and sees you through the winter months with grace and lightness.

Aromatherapy for Winter

During the chill of winter, when the days contract and the cold tightens, finding warmth within becomes a cherished pursuit. Aromatherapy offers a comforting embrace, a method to envelop yourself in tranquillity and warmth through the simple yet profound power of scent. It's an approach both ancient and intuitive, tapping into the invisible threads that connect scent and memory, harnessing them to shape our inner landscapes when the world outside feels dormant and subdued.

The practice of aromatherapy involves the use of essential oils, which are extracted from various plants. These oils capture the very essence of the plants' healing properties, serving as a conduit to balance the body and mind. In the depths of winter, when daylight retreats and chills deepen, leveraging the power of essential oils can provide not only warmth but a sense of wellness and refuge.

Among the myriad of essential oils available, certain ones resonate deeply with the winter season. Think of warming oils like cinnamon, clove, and ginger, which spark an internal fire akin to wrapping oneself in a plush blanket. These scents don't just warm the air; they have the ability to invigorate the spirit, offering both stimulation and comfort. The spicy notes of cinnamon and clove, traditionally associated with winter festivities, bring forth a sense of nostalgia and community, fostering emotional warmth.

Then, there are the grounding oils like cedarwood and sandalwood. These carry a rich, earthy aroma that can anchor your being when the cold winds threaten to unroot your sense of comfort. Cedarwood, with its balsamic undertones, offers a serene base, allowing for deep reflection and introspection, much needed during the contemplative quiet of winter. Similarly, sandalwood acts as a balm for heightened emotions, encouraging relaxation and peacefulness.

For many, winter also means battling the menace of colds and congestion. Here, eucalyptus and peppermint offer relief; their brisk, invigorating scents open the airways and encourage easy breathing. Eucalyptus, with its refreshing, camphorous scent, cuts through congestion, while peppermint provides a cooling sensation that sharpens focus and clarity.

Creating your own aromatic winter sanctuary at home can be an inviting and straightforward process. Diffuse your choice of essential oils in a diffuser, transforming the ambient atmosphere with subtle tendrils of scent. Ultrasonic diffusers are recommended as they blend water and essential oil, sending a fine mist into the air without the need for heat, thus preserving the oils' potent properties.

Alternatively, indulge in a warm, soothing bath enhanced with a few drops of essential oils. When combined with Epsom salts, the oils not only scent the water but also offer muscular relaxation — an excellent remedy after braving the cold outdoors. The combination of heat, water, and aroma creates a multisensory experience that warms both body and mind.

If you're seeking a more hands-on experience, consider creating a personal massage oil blend. Mix a few drops of your preferred essential oil with a carrier oil such as sweet almond or jojoba, and use it to massage your hands, feet, or temples. This practice can fortify your connection to your body, offering grounding energy that counters the winter's encroaching chill.

Aromatherapy need not be confined to the personal realm either. Creating a communal atmosphere with selected scents can enhance shared spaces, inspiring an environment of collective comfort and togetherness. A living room infused with a citrus blend—think sweet orange or bergamot—can uplift and energise, while also serving as a social glue during gatherings.

As with all things, it's crucial to be mindful of the quality of the essential oils you choose. Opt for pure, organic oils when possible, ensuring they are free from synthetic additives. Quality will significantly impact the efficacy and aroma of the oils, rendering the therapeutic experience deeper and more authentic.

Engaging with aromatherapy is more than a pursuit of physical comfort—it's a ritual that can also enhance mental resilience. As the outward silence of winter wraps around us, the inner world benefits immensely from attention and care. Cultivating a routine with essential oils can serve as a touchstone, a tangible reminder of warmth and self-nurturance amidst winter's starkness.

Embrace this practice with gentle curiosity, allowing yourself to explore which scents most intimately resonate with your needs and emotions. The art of aromatherapy is rich and varied, presenting myriad opportunities to discover blends that speak directly to you, balancing and revitalising your spirit as the snow falls around your haven.

Thus, in creating a cozy home environment during the winter months, harnessing the power of aromatherapy is akin to planting a garden of warmth and wellbeing inside your home. It's an invitation to turn inward, to breathe deeply, and to find solace and rejuvenation in the singular embrace of scent. As winter weaves its way through the season, let the fragrances of choice serve as your guide to inner peace and balance, enriching your winter experience with every inhale.

Chapter 4:
Morning Rituals for Inner Warmth

As the dawn light slowly filters through the winter mist, we find ourselves at a threshold of possibilities, where the quietude of the morning offers a unique opportunity to kindle an inner fire that defies the cold. Creating a nurturing morning ritual is about more than routines; it is an art form that weaves together intention and action. From the gentle embrace of a warm cup of herbal tea to a meditative pause, each ritual becomes a thread in the tapestry of our day, infusing it with steadiness and strength. Embrace movement that wakes the body with a tender vibrancy — whether through mindful stretching or a brisk walk amid nature's dormant beauty. As we breathe in the crisp air, we fill our lungs with potential and invite our spirits to awaken. By allowing these rituals to root us in the present, we lay a foundation of resilience that carries us through the winter day, fostering an inner warmth that transcends the chill outside.

Winter Morning Routine

A winter morning holds a certain magic, a quiet invitation to begin the day with intention, cultivating the inner warmth needed to face the world. The first light trickles through frosted windows, casting a gentle glow and inviting you to embrace the stillness before the hustle of the day commences. There's a sort of sacredness to this time, a choice to be made between staying cocooned in the warmth of your bed or stretching your limbs into the chill of the day. It's in these delicate moments that our most cherished rituals are born, rituals that go on to shape our day with grace and vitality.

Each individual's winter morning routine can be seen as a tapestry, woven with threads that resonate with exploration, comfort, and self-care. At the heart of these routines are practices designed to nurture body and mind, ensuring we remain grounded, regardless of the weather outside. Such practices tread the line between tradition and personal preference, drawing on actions that not only invigorate but also soothe.

For many, the day begins with a moment of stillness. It may be meditation, journaling, or simply sitting quietly with a steaming cup of herbal tea. This practice isn't just about pause; it's about creating a space where gratitude and positive intention for the day ahead can flourish. Taking these first moments to breathe deeply encourages a calm and resilient mindset, which is the foundation for tackling any of winter's challenges.

Once you've spent time honouring your mind, it's important to tune in to your body's needs. Physical movement, even the gentlest kind, is a vital aspect of an enriching winter morning routine. A short yoga practice or a series of stretches can awaken your senses and invigorate your muscles, shaking off the stiffness that often accompanies cold nights. As you move, you stoke a fire of energy within, which kindles warmth to your extremities while also fortifying your spirit.

The next chapter of your morning might involve a nourishing breakfast, crafted not simply for sustenance, but with intention. Winter invites us to savour our meals, and breakfast is no exception. Warm, fulfilling dishes like porridge with seasonal fruits or eggs with spices can fortify your body with nutrients and warmth, preparing you to face the crisp air beyond your doorstep. Often, these practices of creating and consuming breakfast provide comfort within the chill, an act of love that sets a nurturing tone for the day.

A ritual that aligns with the rhythm of the season could also include mindful hydration. Simply swapping cold water for warm, infused teas or gentle sips of lemon water can subtly build warmth from within. This act of hydration allows a sense of fluidity, promoting circulation and inviting mental clarity as you step into the hours that follow.

Beyond what we do, there's also the question of how we dress to embrace winter mornings. The choice to envelop yourself in layers, selecting clothing that offers both comfort and functionality, is an act of self-care. Each garment acts not just as a barrier against the cold, but as an expression of care towards yourself, preparing you to meet the day's experiences with resilience.

In cultivating a winter morning routine, it's key to recognise the importance of balance—balancing productivity with relaxation, activity with rest, nourishment with enjoyment. This routine becomes a quietly empowering practice, where even the simplest of actions, performed with presence and intention, build an enduring inner warmth.

Another dimension of a winter morning is the sensory experience it provides. Perhaps your morning is enriched with the gentle hum of a favourite tune or the fragrant embrace of essential oils wafting from a diffuser. These subtle layers add depth to the habitual, turning ordinary moments into extraordinary experiences. The scents and sounds around us influence our mood, and by choosing those that uplift or soothe, we can enhance our connection to the wellbeing we desire during winter months.

Winter mornings may seem daunting with their icy air and muted skies, yet these routines act as a beacon, guiding us through this heightened awareness of the season's qualities. They transform the mundane into meaningful, gelling a personal rhythm that honours both our aspirations and our natural inclinations.

Ultimately, by weaving together elements that resonate personally, the winter morning routine becomes a treasured mosaic of care, reflection, and growth. It is crafted not merely as a checklist of activities but as a living embodiment of what it means to embrace inner warmth when the world outside is anything but. In this way, the routine itself is a practitioner of harmony, dancing between the pressing schedules of modern life and the tranquil embrace of winter's grace.

This winter, consider embracing your morning rituals with renewed intention. Let this grounding sequence be something more than a habit, but a joyful surrender to the subtle joys and invites of winter. Through this, step by step, breath by breath, we cultivate resilience and warmth, inner fires stoked by the choices we make each morning, carrying their glow into the day ahead.

Energising Practices

As the winter dawn nudges you awake, the world outside might be cloaked in a chilly embrace. But inside, you have the potential to awaken a warmth that sets the tone for your day. Energising practices are about purposefully kick-starting your morning so you carry that invigoration through the frosty hours ahead. These routines don't just drive away the remnants of sleep—they reconnect you with a sense of vitality, ensure your spirits are lifted, and keep inner warmth glowing.

While it's often tempting to linger under the covers with an extra snooze in winter's grip, starting the day with physical energy can be transformative. Begin with some gentle stretches right there in bed. Stretch your arms high above your head and point your toes. Feel the life awaken in your muscles, as if telling your body that today is yours to conquer. Stretching not only increases circulation but also helps clear the mind. Inhale slowly, hold it, and exhale, picturing each breath removing the fog of sleep.

Transitioning from the warmth of the bed into the day, let water be your companion. A splash of cold water on the face or a short cool shower not only awakens the skin but also stimulates an increase in alertness. It's an invigorating practice that triggers circulation and provides a natural jolt of energy better than any caffeinated drink. If that seems too jarring, alternating hot and cold water works too, giving the body a gentle wake-up call without the shock of an icy blast.

Although the physiological responses are crucial, energising practices extend beyond the physical. Engage your mind with a mindfulness moment. Sit quietly and set an intention for the day or practice mindfulness meditation. Keep this simple; it could be a minute or two, focusing solely on your breath. Let your thoughts drift by without holding onto them like a leaf floating on a stream. This practice not only cultivates stillness but also focuses the mind, providing a steady foundation for the day's challenges.

Winter light can seem scarce, and those grey mornings often crave colour and vibrancy. Consider bringing more light into your mornings by practising sun salutations. Even if it's dim outside, these yoga sequences stimulate the body, synchronise your movement with breath, and boost your endorphin levels, which in turn aids in counteracting the winter blues.

Music is another excellent source of energy. Create a playlist of songs that inspire movement and joy. Use it as a backdrop to your morning routine, allowing your body to sway to the rhythm as you prepare breakfast or get dressed. Music has a unique ability to uplift and energise, tapping into emotional reserves that might feel dulled in winter.

However, energy isn't only about physical or sensory stimulation—it's also about nutrition. Fuel your body with food that burns slow and steady like a log fire. Energising breakfasts in winter could include oats, nuts, berries, and a touch of honey to start the metabolic fire. A warm bowl of porridge sprinkled with cinnamon can feel like a hug from the inside.

As you eat, practice mindful eating. Appreciating each bite nurtures the spirit, allowing you to savour flavours while also tuning into the body's nutritional needs, creating a more fulfilling and energising experience. Sip on a warming cup of herbal tea, rich in herbs that stimulate and invigorate. Ginger or peppermint tea can work wonders to awaken the senses.

After preparing your body, connect it with the earth. Maybe it's a brief walk through a frosty garden or merely standing outside for a moment, breathing in the crisp air. Notice the contrasts—the crunch of snow or frost, the stillness of a barren tree, or the warmth the sun still manages to spread. This short communion with nature can be absorbing and energising, providing a different kind of fuel that makes you feel more grounded and alive.

In the quiet of winter mornings, when activity beyond your door seems frozen, energising practices offer the promise of warmth and vitality. They present the opportunity to build resilience, to bolster your spirit against the cold. By thoughtfully incorporating these routines, you can ignite an inner fire that will not just propel you through your mornings but carry through your days.

These practices may seem small, but they're acts of self-care—precious investments in well-being that cultivate a deeper connection with yourself. Embrace them with openness and give yourself every reason to move forward with a heartfelt conviction that, even in the coldest months, warmth is never out of reach.

Chapter 5:
Embracing Outdoor Activities

When the world is draped in winter's cloak, stepping outside might seem daunting, yet it's where true revitalisation awaits. The crisp air invigorates, and beneath the crunch of frost underfoot lies a profound connection to nature's quiet resilience. Embracing outdoor activities, even in shorter daylight hours, empowers you to break free from the confines of winter's hibernation. Whether it's the simple pleasure of a winter walk or the invigorating challenge of safe outdoor exercise, each moment spent outside nurtures your well-being. By revelling in the rhythmic cadence of your breath coalescing with the refreshing chill, you unlock an inner warmth that nourishes both body and soul. Here, amidst the stillness, you find energy, clarity, and the gentle reminder that winter, too, is a time for growth and renewal.

Winter Walks

In the cold embrace of winter, when daylight is brief and the chill can be sharp, stepping outside might not be the first thing on our minds. Yet there lies a hidden charm in winter walks. It's in these quiet yet invigorating moments that we can truly embrace the season and find connections to our inner warmth. Think of a winter walk as a meditative practice, one that reawakens the senses dulled by the daily grind.

The world feels different under a gentle snowfall or glistening frost. As we set out, each step becomes a deliberate action, our breath visible in the cold air serving as a rhythmic guide. The unique tranquillity of a snow-covered landscape offers a fresh perspective. It clears away the clutter of thoughts, leaving room for contemplation and peace. Everything slows down; the hustle of summer months is replaced with the slow, deliberate pace of winter.

Winter walks are not just for the soul, though—they're a balm for the body as well. The cool air invigorates our systems, prompting circulation, and boosting physical energy levels. There's something about braving the elements and feeling the crisp air on our faces that invigorates more than the body; it stirs the spirit. This is where the motivational force lies, in that marriage of simplicity and rejuvenation that only a walk in winter can provide.

Venturing out may initially seem daunting, especially when the environment calls for comfort and warmth indoors. However, preparing for a winter walk is an exercise in mindfulness. Consider the layers of clothing, each carefully chosen to shield and insulate. Think of it as armouring oneself for intimate time with nature's quieter but still vibrant face. Gloves, hats, and scarves aren't just practical tools; they're the embodiments of self-care. Choosing them becomes a ritual, one that signifies the readiness to engage deeply with the season.

Once enveloped in the outdoors, notice the crunch of the snow beneath your boots, the intricate designs of ice on windows, the stark silhouettes of bare trees against a pale sky. Nature, stripped of its traditional aesthetic, reveals its subtler charms. Here, minimalism reigns supreme, and with it, an opportunity to marvel at the small details you might otherwise overlook. Each step peels back layers of worry and, in their place, instils clarity and peace.

Encountering winter wildlife can be another unexpected joy. Hardy robins, brightly coloured in contrast to their muted surroundings, remind us of resilience. Spotting a lone rabbit or a cluster of tiny footprints in the snow speaks of life's continuation despite the harshness. The echoes of these sights linger within, encouraging the same persistence and adaptability as these creatures, reinforcing our own resilience in challenging times.

The serenity of a winter walk also offers a fertile ground for reflection. It's in the rhythm of walking, the gentle cadence of movement blending with thought, that we find introspection. The world, covered in blankets of white, symbolises a blank canvas, encouraging us to consider our own paths and the marks we wish to leave. The landscape transforms into a metaphor for personal growth and renewal, no matter the season or how dormant things may seem.

For those with a creative bent, these walks can stir inspiration. The stillness, the contrast, and the transformation of familiar settings under the snow invite new ways of thinking. There's an added layer of creativity in the act of capturing these moments, be it through photography, writing, or simply storing them in the mind's eye. Allow the purity of these experiences to influence your creative processes.

Sometimes, a walk with a friend or companion can enhance the experience. Share in the tranquillity, exchange thoughts, yet remain keenly aware of the shared silence that winter imposes. Conversing in the open air, with faces flushed by the cold, nurtures social bonds. Winter walks can turn into cherished communal rituals, adding richness to social experiences during these more isolated months.

Paths that cut through woodlands, sprawling parks glistening with morning frost, or even snow-draped city streets are more than routes to traverse. They're avenues to commune with nature and the self. The realisation that every journey is unique and that even the same path walked twice can offer a vastly different experience is both humbling and exciting.

Upon returning home, the contrast between the cold exterior world and the warm embrace of a heated room is deliciously comforting. It's this juxtaposition that truly defines the joy of a winter walk—the knowledge that comfort is available at the end brings a profound sense of gratitude and satisfaction. This transition from the brisk vitality of the outdoors to the snug contentment of indoors allows us to appreciate each aspect more fully.

Winter walks are an invitation to explore beyond the superficial layers of the season, encouraging an embrace of deeper connections, be it within ourselves or the environment. They offer a chance to engage with winter's more subtle beauty and emerge with a refreshed sense of well-being and a fortified spirit. In taking those deliberate steps into the heart of winter, one uncovers layers of insight and resilience, warming the spirit and invigorating the soul, regardless of the chill.

Safe Outdoor Exercise

Immersing oneself in the brisk embrace of winter can be an invigorating experience. As the chill bites the air, it awakens a vivacious spirit, reminding us that outdoor activities can be as enriching in winter as they are during the balmier seasons. Exercising safely in the outdoors during this time not only enhances physical health but also revitalises the mind and spirit, offering a unique blend of challenges and rewards that are deeply fulfilling.

Venture into the winter landscape with an open heart, noticing the transformation that occurs as everything is covered with a glistening sheath. It's crucial, however, to approach outdoor exercise with mindfulness, preparing adequately to make the most of the invigorating cold while staying safe. Dressing in layers is an essential strategy; it allows you to adjust your clothing to the varying intensity of your workout and external temperatures. Opt for moisture-wicking fabrics close to your skin to keep dry, as the combination of moisture and cold air can make you feel colder. Further layers should provide insulation, with an outer layer that protects against wind and moisture.

As you step out into the crisp air, your choice of footwear becomes paramount. Selecting shoes with good grip can help prevent slips on wet or icy surfaces, ensuring each stride is firm and confident. If snow is abundant where you live, snowshoes or trail boots with spikes might offer the best protection and stability. Attentiveness to path conditions allows you to choose routes that maintain safety, while still offering the breathtaking views and serenity that winter landscapes provide.

Before embarking on any vigorous activity, warming up your muscles is vital to prevent injury. A proper warm-up raises your body temperature and increases blood flow to crucial muscle groups, readying your body for more dynamic movements. Simple exercises like jumping jacks or a brisk walk are effective ways to start, especially when the temperatures plummet. Stretching post-exercise, especially while still warm, can further help in maintaining flexibility and reducing muscle soreness.

Hydration is often overlooked in winter, mistaking the cool air for a lack of dehydration risk. However, the body's need for fluids remains constant, regardless of the season. Ensuring you drink water before, during, and after exercise is crucial in maintaining energy levels and aiding recovery. A thermos of warm water or herbal tea can be a comforting and practical companion on a chilly day.

Listening to your body is another cornerstone of safe outdoor exercise. The cool temperatures require a nuanced understanding of your physical limits. Pay attention to signs of cold-related distress like numbness, fatigue, or shivering, and respond promptly by adjusting your activity level, clothing, or seeking shelter if necessary. It's about finding balance, ensuring exertion doesn't edge into discomfort or risk.

The winter environment, with its stark beauty, offers a perfect backdrop for embracing exercises that invigorate both body and soul. Winter walking, particularly in natural settings, can be a meditative practice, inviting tranquility and clarity. Ingenuous movements, like yoga or tai chi, can also adapt beautifully to an outdoor winter routine, especially when performed in quiet parks or natural reserves, where the peace of nature inspires introspection and grounding.

For those who wish for a more structured routine, engaging in winter sports like cross-country skiing or ice skating can be both exhilarating and enriching. The rhythmic motion of skiing along snow-draped trails offers a full-body workout that strengthens cardiovascular health, enhances endurance, and provides a profound sense of freedom. Ice skating, similarly, builds core strength and coordination, whisking you into a dreamy dance across the ice. Both these activities require respect for the conditions, ensuring equipment is in good repair and that local safety guidelines are adhered to.

Group activities and clubs can make winter exercise a social pursuit, adding motivation and encouragement. Outdoor meetups for running, cycling, or hiking are opportunities to share the winter landscape with others, fostering camaraderie and shared joy in the cold. What better way to relish the season than alongside like-minded individuals embracing the chill?

Safety isn't just physical; mental readiness is also key. Preparing oneself with a positive mindset frames the experience, allowing challenges presented by winter's unpredictability to be approached with curiosity rather than hesitation. Equip yourself with tools for mental resilience—perhaps a mantra or an anticipated reward post-exercise—fueling motivation on even the greyest of days.

Additionally, technology can be a valuable ally. Apps and wearable devices can help track your exercises and monitor weather conditions, ensuring your safety and enhancing your winter adventure. Always inform someone of your plans, particularly if you're venturing into secluded areas, and carry a small safety kit including essentials such as a whistle, first aid supplies, and a thermal blanket for emergencies.

Lastly, never underestimate the environment's capacity to surprise and delight. Each day brings new wonders, the immaculate beauty of frosted landscapes, and the crispness of fresh snow underfoot. By engaging with this season's rhythm, you'll uncover the multifarious benefits that safe outdoor exercise can bestow, creating a vibrant, resilient self, tuned to the serene yet invigorating melody of winter.

Chapter 6:
Winter Skincare and Bodycare

As the chill of winter wraps around us, our skin often bears the brunt of harsh winds and biting cold. It cries out for nurturing and protection, not unlike our spirits that crave warmth and comfort in these months. This chapter unveils rituals and practices that invite not just lotion and oils, but also a deeper connection with oneself. Enveloping your skin in rich, hydrating layers can be an act of self-love, echoing the care we give to our inner world. A nourishing winter bath can transform into a sacred retreat, with every drop of essential oil offering solace and serenity. Embrace this season as an opportunity to cherish your skin and soul, aligning your bodycare rituals with the profound need for inner balance. Each step in this self-care journey is an invitation to connect with your body, honouring its resilience and cherishing its role as your steadfast companion through winter's embrace.

Protecting Your Skin

As the winds of winter begin to whisper and temperatures take a plunge, protecting your skin becomes essential. The harsh combination of cold air outdoors and dry warmth indoors often leaves our skin parched and vulnerable, requiring us to take deliberate steps to maintain its health and vitality. By nurturing it correctly, we can shield it from the adverse impacts of winter and unveil a glow that exudes warmth and health throughout the season.

One of the first elements to examine is your cleanser. During winter, consider switching to a gentler, more hydrating formula. Harsh cleansers tend to strip the skin of its natural oils, leaving it dehydrated. Opt for a cream-based or oil-based cleanser that cleans effectively while preserving moisture. These types of cleansers not only cleanse but also add a layer of protection from the unforgiving elements. After all, in winter, hydration is not just a luxury; it's an absolute necessity.

Moisturising often serves as the cornerstone of any winter skincare routine. The air's low humidity level necessitates a richer, more emollient moisturiser compared to what you might prefer during the warmer months. Ingredients like hyaluronic acid, glycerin, and ceramides work wonders in drawing moisture into the skin and sealing it in. It's also worth considering products containing natural oils, such as argan, jojoba, or almond oil, which provide additional nourishment and create a barrier against environmental stressors.

Exfoliation, while still crucial, requires a more cautious approach in winter. Over-exfoliating can lead to irritation and sensitivity. Instead of daily exfoliation, consider doing it once or twice a week with a gentle exfoliator. This will help remove dead skin cells that can create a dull appearance, allowing moisturisers and other treatments to work more effectively. Think of it as preparing the canvas so that all the nourishing paint can be absorbed beautifully.

We mustn't overlook the role of a diligent and thoughtful night routine in protecting our skin. As we rest, the skin enters repair mode, making it an ideal time to apply treatments that might be too heavy for daytime wear. Using a nourishing night cream or overnight mask can make a significant difference. Ingredients such as peptides and antioxidants like vitamin C can help in repairing and regenerating the skin from what the elements have worn away during the day.

Also, protect your skin by embracing hydration from the inside out. Aim to consume more fluids than you might feel inclined to in the colder months. Herbal teas, infused waters, and warm soups can contribute to the skin's hydration and well-being. Supplementing your diet with essential fatty acids, found in fish or flaxseed oil, can enhance skin's suppleness and resilience from within.

While the sun might feel distant, don't abandon your SPF. Harmful UV rays penetrate even through cloudy skies and can reflect off snow, causing skin damage. Sunscreen should remain a staple in your skincare armoury throughout the year. A good practice is to apply a moisturiser that combines SPF protection, merging two vital steps into one for those brisk winter mornings.

Humidity levels in your home can also have a profound impact on your skin's moisture levels. This is where the quiet hum of a humidifier becomes invaluable. By increasing the moisture in the air, a humidifier can prevent your skin from resembling the parched landscapes of winter. Place one in your bedroom or workspace, wherever you spend substantial time, to keep your environment, and consequently your skin, more balanced.

But it's not just your face that needs safeguarding. Remember that your hands and lips are also exposed to the elements. Use a moisturising hand cream frequently, especially after washing your hands, and keep lip balm handy to stave off chapping and cracking. Prevention is always more effective and pleasant than trying to remedy an existing problem.

Finally, listen to what your skin is trying to tell you. Winter skincare is not about covering every inch with products, but rather about understanding and responding to your skin's needs. If your skin feels tight or looks dull, it could be asking for more hydration or a break from certain products. Let intuition guide you as you sort through the many options and suggestions.

By taking these steps to protect your skin during the winter months, you construct a resilient, nurturing routine that supports not just your outer glow but a profound inner warmth. As you embrace these practices, the season's chill transforms from an adversary to an opportunity for care, reminding us of our capacity to thrive, even in the coldest times. More than keeping our skin safe, it's about honouring our body's largest organ with love and respect, day by day, throughout the season.

Winter Bath Rituals

In the heart of winter, as the world outside shivers beneath a blanket of frost and snow, there's a moment of peace and warmth waiting to be found in the simple embrace of a bath. Winter bath rituals offer not just warmth, but a holistic sanctuary for both body and mind. The ritual of bathing in winter is an opportunity to pause, reflect, and replenish our energies, embracing the season's quietude and using it to nurture inner balance.

Winter baths can be infused with intention and purpose, creating an experience that transcends mere hygiene. The first step to an enriching bath ritual is setting the scene. Dim the lights and perhaps even light a few candles, moments like these deserve the soft, warm glow that only candlelight can offer. Aromatherapy plays a key role here; the scents of lavender, eucalyptus, or sandalwood can transform a simple bath into a fragrant escape.

But it's not just about the smells. Bath art perhaps, allows us to explore enriching the bathwater itself. Salts such as Epsom or Himalayan pink add minerals and help relax tired and aching muscles. Essential oils can be dropped sparingly, bringing their therapeutic properties directly to the bath. A few drops of rose oil are enough to soothe the skin, lead to a lighter mood, and leave you feeling enveloped in luxury. As your body unwinds in the warm water, the tension in your muscles begins to dissolve, and with it, the worries of the day.

Consider incorporating herbs into your bath to enhance its healing properties. A mesh bag filled with chamomile flowers or green tea can do wonders for your skin, leaving it feeling soft and hydrated. These ingredients not only have topical benefits but also offer aromatic ones that can calm your mind, making your bath a truly restorative experience.

Beyond selecting the right ingredients, mindfulness is the keystone of a winter bath ritual. As you soak, take deep, deliberate breaths. Feel the steam on your face, focus on the gentle ripple of water against your skin, and centre yourself in the present moment. It's in these moments that we realise the true power of a moment of stillness amid the busyness of life. Our minds can race with the demands of the external world, yet in this sanctuary, they find respite.

Varying the temperature of your bath can introduce a new level of therapeutic benefit. While the end goal is to soak in warmth, consider starting with a quick, invigorating rinse with cooler water. This practice, known as contrast hydrotherapy, is believed to stimulate the immune system, improve circulation, and invigorate one's spirit.

For a deeper spiritual dimension, one might choose to incorporate guided visualisation or meditation practices into the bath. The warmth of the water can deepen the meditative state, helping ease you into a tranquil mindset where you might visualise letting go of stress with each exhalation, sensing peace wash over you with each inhale.

After your body feels completely relaxed, and all your worries seem to float away with the steam, gently transition out of the tub. Pat your skin dry with a towel to preserve its warmth and moisture. Then, massage nourishing oils or lotions onto your skin, sealing in the soft, refreshed feeling that a good bath instills.

And don't rush this conclusion. Wrap a fluffy robe around you, savouring the comfort and protection it offers against the brisk air beyond the bathroom sanctuary. Allow yourself to linger in the moment, perhaps with a cup of herbal tea to extend the ritual beyond the bath.

The benefits of winter bath rituals are myriad, going well beyond clean skin to encompass the rejuvenation of one's spirit and emotional well-being. It's not merely water in which you soak, but the gentle embrace of an ancient and deeply personal practice for warming the soul in the coldest of seasons.

In this timeless tradition of water and warmth, we find more than temporary physical relief; we discover enduring emotional resilience. As the chill of winter surrounds, the warmth of these rituals becomes not just a comfort, but a lifelong embrace of self-care and renewal.

Chapter 7:
Mental Resilience in the Cold Months

The cold months can weigh heavily on the mind, but building mental resilience during this time is both essential and empowering. As the world outside becomes a tapestry of grey and white, the mind can be a vibrant counterpoint, an inner sanctuary of warmth and vitality. It's about embracing a mindset that thrives on adaptability, letting each breath anchor you in the present. This season invites introspection, allowing space to cultivate a practice of mindful meditation and a positive mindset. Just as trees stand firm through winter snow, drawing strength from silent roots, we too can ground ourselves in stillness, drawing from our deepest reserves of positivity. Engaging regularly in mindful practices helps to soften the stark edges of winter's chill, transforming them into opportunities for growth and self-discovery. By nurturing a resilient spirit, you not only weather the cold months but flourish within them, discovering an unexpected warmth in the embrace of winter's quietude.

Mindful Meditation

The chill of winter can often seep into our bones, not just physically but mentally as well. In these months, when the sun appears only briefly and the landscapes are painted in shades of grey and white, the practice of mindful meditation becomes a beacon of warmth and tranquillity. It invites us to journey inward, finding calm and resilience amidst the outer cold.

Mindful meditation is about engaging with each moment fully, recognising it without judging or attempting to change it. It offers a sanctuary for the mind, a gentle refuge from the harshness of winter's touch. As we sit in stillness, we create space for the mind to rest and our thoughts to settle, much like snowflakes drifting softly to the ground.

Incorporating meditation into your winter routine might initially seem daunting. However, it can be as simple as finding a comfortable spot in your home, perhaps by a window where the daylight casts a soft glow. Close your eyes, take several deep breaths and let the awareness of your breath anchor you to the present moment. Feel the simplicity of breathing and how it connects you to life.

Variety can enhance your meditation practice. One day, focus on your breath's rhythm. Another, tune into the subtle sensations within your body, gently observing areas of tension and warmth. Winter's tranquillity may inspire you to engage in visualisation exercises, such as imagining yourself surrounded by a serene, snowy landscape where each breath melts away stress.

Winter's quiet invites reflection, making this season an exceptional time for meditative practice. It's a period to acknowledge the past, embrace the present, and softly contemplate the future. Mindful meditation encourages this reflection without getting lost in a whirlwind of thoughts; it's about observing feelings and thoughts as they arise and gently letting them go.

With regular meditation, you'll find a sense of inner warmth growing. The practice builds resilience not by shielding us from life's challenges but by empowering us to face them with clarity and calm. It's like wrapping a soft, warm blanket around your mind, preparing it to withstand the chill of winter stressors and discomforts.

Many find it helpful to journal after meditating. Writing down insights garnered during meditation can solidify and extend the sense of clarity and peace achieved. Whether it's a sentence or a page, this written reflection can serve as a reminder of your journey and progress as you move through the colder months.

Meditating with others can also deepen this practice. While winter may isolate us physically, mindful meditation can bridge distances. Consider joining a meditation group or participating in an online session to share energy and experiences, fostering a sense of community and support. Sharing this journey amplifies its effects, aiding mutual growth and understanding.

Sound is an ally in mindful meditation. The use of gentle music or nature sounds—like rainfall or crackling firewood—can ground the mind and make the experience more immersive. As you enter this soothing auditory landscape, it becomes easier to focus and let go of the clutter that frequently invades our thoughts.

The beauty of mindful meditation lies in its adaptability and personalisation. There are numerous styles to experiment with: from loving-kindness meditation, which fosters empathy and compassion, to body scan meditation, which enhances awareness of bodily sensations. Embrace a trial-and-error approach to find what resonates most and cultivates the deepest sense of calm within you.

As the winter days stretch on and the nights draw near, mindful meditation becomes an essential practice in nurturing our mental resilience. It's a repetitive yet rewarding cycle of coming home to ourselves, creating warmth and light within that echoes outward. With dedication and openness, meditation can transform the way we experience winter, filling the coldest months with peace and profound insight.

In conclusion, let mindful meditation be your steadfast companion this winter. Allow its gentle power to ground you, connecting you to an inner fortitude that matches the beauty and quiet strength of the season itself. The path inward is deeply personal, yet it aligns us with a universal rhythm, a shared human striving for peace amid life's inevitable tumult and chill. Through this practice, you can cultivate not just survival but a flourishing resilience and warmth, bringing light even into the darkest days of winter.

Building a Positive Mindset

As the chill of winter settles in, fostering a positive mindset becomes both a challenge and an opportunity. The cold months naturally prompt a retreat into our homes, and often, into our thoughts. This season invites introspection, but with it can come a heaviness that many recognise as winter blues. To cultivate a positive mindset during this time, it's pivotal to embrace practices that enliven and uplift the spirit, transforming this introspective season into a time of growth and resilience.

Consider the power of gratitude. Even in the face of dreary weather, the simple act of acknowledging what you're thankful for can instil a profound sense of positivity. Start each day consciously noting three things you appreciate. These could be as grand as a supportive network of friends, or as simple as that first sip of comforting tea. Gratitude, in its gentle yet powerful way, shifts focus from what's lacking to what's abundant, infusing each day with a sense of blessing and fulfilment.

Visualisation, too, can be an effective ally. By imagining positive outcomes and envisioning oneself navigating the colder months with ease and joy, you enhance your mental resilience. Picture a warm, inviting scene: yourself nestled by a fire, a blanket draped over your knees, a book in hand. Such images can serve as mental check-ins that remind you of your own capabilities and the joys yet to come. This mental rehearsal fortifies your mind and prepares it to focus on creating a reality that mirrors these positive scenarios.

It's valuable to acknowledge that negativity often flourishes in isolation. Counter this by surrounding yourself with positivity. Whether it's through music, literature, or social connections, immerse yourself in experiences and environments that inspire and elevate you. A well-curated winter playlist, filled with tunes that speak to the heart, keeps spirits high and counters the desolate silence that sometimes accompanies long winter nights. Similarly, books penned with warmth and wisdom offer perspectives that expand and enrich the mind.

Furthermore, practising acceptance is essential. Winter, with its shorter days and extended darkness, teaches us about the cyclical nature of life. Accepting what is beyond our control, instead of resisting or resenting it, can significantly alleviate mental burdens. Embrace each day's unique rhythm, understanding that this season is just one part of a larger cycle. Acceptance alleviates pressure, paving the way for peace and a clearer focus on what can be influenced and transformed.

Positive affirmations, used consistently, can rewire thought patterns, embedding optimistic perspectives in the subconscious mind. Each morning, or as part of a bedtime ritual, reaffirm your strengths and your potential to thrive within the winter months. Words have power, and repeated affirmations serve to anchor your capabilities and intentions, weaving positivity into the very fabric of your lived experience.

Mindfulness also plays a pivotal role in developing a resilient mindset. By staying present, fully engaging with each moment, one can prevent the mind from wandering into peaks of anxiety or valleys of despondency. Engage in daily mindfulness exercises. Feel the crisp air biting playfully at your cheeks during a morning walk or savour the taste of a warm meal prepared with care. Such practices ground you in reality, enabling a focused, calm approach to the day's challenges.

The act of setting realistic goals propels the mind forward with purpose. Winter's more confined nature is perfect for small, manageable projects that yield satisfaction upon completion. This sense of achievement fuels positive emotions and sets the groundwork for ongoing self-improvement, reinforcing a belief in one's capability to thrive in any circumstance. Celebrate each accomplishment, no matter how minor, as these victories accumulate into significant personal growth.

Remember, nurturing a positive mindset extends to how we cope with challenging emotions. It's okay to feel sadness or frustration brought by winter's constraints. Instead of suppressing these feelings, observe them, understand their origins, and allow them to pass. Like leaves caught in a gentle breeze, emotions are transient and shift with time. By permitting yourself to feel all facets of your emotional spectrum, you deal with them constructively rather than letting them take root.

Social connections can be a wellspring of positivity. During winter, these relationships can lend warmth and support, pulling you from solitude into shared laughter and mutual support. Engage in simple shared activities, whether it's cooking a meal together or exchanging thoughts over a virtual call. These interactions remind us of the bonds that surpass any seasonal limitations and the joy inherent in companionship.

Lastly, consider the transformative power of creativity. Engaging in creative activities stimulates the mind and offers a channel for expressing and processing emotions. Whether through painting, knitting, or any form of artistic expression, creativity not only distracts from negative thinking but builds a foundation of joy and accomplishment. In bringing something new into the world, no matter how small, you contribute to a narrative of optimism and endless potential.

Amid winter's demands, the journey to a positive mindset is deeply personal yet universally relevant. By integrating these practices into daily life, the cold months transform into a crucible for inner strength, where resilience is not only built but thrived upon. Winter's cold cannot erode the internal warmth generated by a positive mindset, a bright fire that sustains and enriches in any season.

Chapter 8:
Social Connections and Winter Wellness

A mid the frosty embrace of winter, nurturing social connections can be a beacon of warmth, enhancing both emotional and physical wellness. As the days grow shorter and the chill deepens, fostering relationships becomes crucial, offering a space where hearts can share stories, laughter, and the simple joy of togetherness. A gathering with friends or family, adorned with creativity and thoughtful touches, can transform a simple get-together into a beloved ritual, strengthening bonds and lifting spirits. These moments of connection counteract the isolation that often creeps in during this season, reminding us that shared warmth and kindness can thaw even the coldest days. Engage in activities that bring people together—from a cosy book club meeting to preparing a meal as a collective effort. Such gatherings not only boost our mental resilience but also instil a sense of belonging, cultivating an enduring inner warmth that transcends the winter months.

Nurturing Relationships

As the days grow shorter and the nights colder, our instinct might be to withdraw into the comforting cocoon of solitude. Yet, this season offers a unique opportunity to nurture the relationships that sustain us. When the outside world is stark and stripped bare, the warmth of human connection becomes more vital than ever. The bonds we share

are like robust fibres of an intricate tapestry, providing richness and resilience to the fabric of our lives.

Winter, with its challenges and charms, encourages reflection—a perfect backdrop for fostering deeper connections with those around us. Whether it's family, friends, or our broader community, these relationships can be a wellspring of support and joy. Research consistently highlights that social connections improve mental health and even physical well-being. In winter, this can be an antidote to the blues that the colder months sometimes bring.

Central to nurturing relationships is presence. In today's fast-paced world, truly being present with others can feel like a luxury. But imagine the impact of a conversation undistracted by screens, where you're fully engaged, listening intently to the thoughts, dreams, and concerns of a loved one. Such moments are not just about exchanging words but about sharing your energy and attention, fostering a space where intimacy can thrive.

The Danish concept of "hygge," often associated with coziness, extends beyond an atmosphere of warmth. It invites us to cherish simple pleasures and cultivate meaningful interactions. Imagine gathering around a table for an evening meal with those who matter, the clinking of cutlery punctuated by laughter. The beauty of these gatherings, no matter how modest, lies in their ability to reinforce the bonds that link us all.

Winter can also be a time to mend estranged relationships. The overarching theme of renewal and reflection invites us to reconsider and reach out. This may take courage, but the rewards are worth it. A heartfelt apology, a gesture of goodwill, or simply extending an olive branch can all pave the way for healing, bringing a sense of peace and closure.

Nurturing relationships during the winter months doesn't always have to happen in person. The digital world offers us tools to maintain connections, no matter the physical distance. Virtual meetings, voice calls, or even a well-thought-out message can remind others that they're valued. A note about something funny or touching—a shared memory perhaps—might brighten someone's day more than you'd imagine.

Moreover, relationships are not only about what we gain but also what we give. Acts of kindness, no matter how small, can strengthen connections and improve our own well-being. A warm meal shared, a small gift given, or simply lending an ear to listen can have a profound impact. It's the notion that giving truly is receiving. Winter, with its emphasis on coming together, invites us to embody this spirit of generosity.

For those exploring spirituality, winter can be a profound time for extending grace and compassion to others. Spiritual teachings across cultures and faiths highlight the importance of love and community as pillars of a fulfilling life. Embracing this can lead to enriched relationships. Consider setting aside a few moments to meditate on the well-being of others, offering prayers or thoughts of compassion, helping you feel more connected to the greater whole.

Additionally, creativity can be an unexpected ally in nurturing relationships. Engaging in collaborative activities or projects with loved ones can fortify bonds and create lasting memories. Whether it's cooking together, embarking on a crafting endeavour, or even building a snowman, shared experiences promote teamwork and understanding. Creativity becomes a bridge, shortening the emotional distances that may have crept in unnoticed.

There's also profound value in recognising and adapting to the changing dynamics within our relationships. Just as winter teaches us about transformation, relationships too evolve with time. We can navigate these changes by embracing open communication and understanding. This adaptability not only strengthens our connections but also enriches our personal growth.

Finally, let's not overlook the relationship we have with ourselves. Self-love and compassion are foundational; nurturing this inner relationship equips us to be more present and loving with others. Winter encourages introspection. Love yourself by setting aside time to understand your needs and desires. In doing so, you're better positioned to nurture and sustain the relationships that matter most.

Nurturing relationships against the backdrop of winter's chill is about more than keeping warm. It's an opportunity to cultivate a deeply interconnected existence with family, friends, and indeed, all beings. As we invest time and effort into nurturing these bonds, we create a tapestry woven with shared love, laughter, and life itself. That tapestry offers warmth against the coldest nights, reminding us that we are, indeed, never truly alone.

Creative Gatherings

In the heart of winter, when days are shorter and the world outside often presents a monochrome tableau, the warmth and vitality of social connections can bring a burst of colour to the monotony. Creative gatherings, in this frosty season, serve as essential sanctuaries where individuals can foster connections, share imaginings, and weave dreams into reality. They're environments where creativity and camaraderie coalesce, crafting a climate of warmth and inspiration that transcends the chill outside.

One of the most rewarding aspects of winter is its inherent quietude, offering a beautiful backdrop for intimate gatherings that cultivate creative expression. Whether around a crackling fireplace or in a cozy living room filled with soft textures and ambient lighting, these encounters can be both soul-nourishing and inspiring. It's in the setting of a creative gathering that people can share laughter, stories, and ideas, igniting both personal and collective creativity. These are places of refuge where imaginations are set free.

Imagine a room filled with friends, warmed by the glow of candles and the sound of gentle music. This idyllic scene becomes the perfect incubator for creativity. Each person brings their own unique flair, contributing to an atmosphere that's both stimulating and soothing. The tactile pleasures of knitting circles, the focused energy of writing workshops, or the collaborative spirit of a group painting session—in these spaces, creativity and connection flourish hand-in-hand. This synergy fosters not only artistic expression but emotional well-being as well.

For those with a penchant for the culinary arts, a shared cooking experience can be particularly enriching. A kitchen bustling with activity, fragrant with the spices of the season, offers a dynamic and sensory-rich space for social creativity. Friends and loved ones gather to create a meal, blending ingredients and ideas, and enjoying the fruits of their labour together. It's a delightful way to combine nourishment, creativity, and connection, celebrating the simple yet profound pleasure of a shared table.

Creative gatherings also offer an opportunity to establish new rituals and traditions that can be carried beyond the winter months. Book clubs, crafting clans, and music circles are all ways to foster community and creativity. These gatherings might be initiated as a response to winter's insularity but can evolve into cherished year-round activities. The power of such communities lies in their ability to not only combat the isolation that winter can bring but to create enduring bonds grounded in creative collaboration.

Some gatherings embrace technology to bridge distances, allowing for virtual creativity. Online workshops and discussion groups can offer similar joy and connection, breaking the boundaries of geography. Whether sharing poetry, discussing a novel, or even participating in a virtual art class, technology provides endless possibilities for staying connected. In these digital spaces, creative exchanges remain vibrant, confirming that the need for human connection transcends the physical realm.

Crafting a personal winter retreat for a group gathering can set the stage for rejuvenation and inspiration. When the environment is thoughtfully designed, it welcomes a mindset open to creative expression. Think of your space as a blank canvas, ready to be adorned with colours, textures, and scents that evoke a sense of peace and possibility. The aesthetic pleasure and sensory richness of a well-curated space can amplify creative energies, inviting inspiration and fostering a nourishing environment for all.

Hosting themed events, like a vintage movie night, a poetry reading club, or a mini art exhibition, can also spark creativity. These themes serve as focal points, offering attendees a shared interest that encourages participation and enhances the sense of community. By establishing a central theme, hosts provide structure to the creative endeavor while allowing free flow of ideas and interaction.

An essential factor in successful creative gatherings is the openness to spontaneity. While a certain level of planning helps create a cohesive event, leaving room for impromptu activities and discussions can often lead to unexpected and delightful results. Spontaneous dance, impromptu music-making, or a sudden storytelling session can create bonds and memories that are cherished long after the ice melts and spring appears.

The role of a facilitator in these gatherings can't be understated. A good host doesn't only manage logistics but also nurtures an inclusive atmosphere where every participant feels valued and heard. Gentle guidance can help weave conversations, ensuring that everyone gets a chance to share their creativity. The facilitator fosters an environment where vulnerability is embraced, encouraging participants to step outside their comfort zones and try new creative practices.

For those who might feel hesitant, stepping into a group setting can sometimes feel daunting. It's worth remembering that creative gatherings thrive on diversity of thought and experience. Everyone has something unique to offer, and even the act of listening can contribute to the creative energy of the group. Curiosity, openness, and the willingness to engage without preconceived notions often bring about the most meaningful experiences.

As the world outside hibernates, creative gatherings illuminate the winter months with the warmth of human connection and the spark of shared creativity. They provide a powerful antidote to the isolation sometimes felt during this season, offering a reminder of our innate need for connection and expression. Each gathering is an opportunity to create, to connect, and to carry the spirit of togetherness beyond the confines of the present moment.

So, as snowflakes begin their delicate descent, and the world wears a coat of white, let us gather in creativity, crafting spaces where warmth is shared, dreams are kindled, and friendships are forged in the glow of shared experience. Through these creative gatherings, we discover not only the vibrant tapestry of others' lives but also the threads that weave our own stories into the wider community.

Chapter 9:
Herbal Remedies for Winter Health

As winter's chill sets in, turning to nature's apothecary offers a nurturing way to bolster our well-being. Herbal remedies provide not just physical sustenance, but also a comforting ritual that ties us to ancient wisdom. Delicate yet potent, herbs like echinacea and elderberry have been used for generations to support the immune system against the stark challenges of the cold months. Crafting herbal teas and tonics becomes an act of self-care, steeped in both tradition and personal intent. With each soothing sip, these concoctions invite warmth from within, fostering a tranquil resilience that sustains us. Embrace the calming power of chamomile or the invigorating zest of ginger, letting these botanical allies guide you through the winter in a way that feels timeless and deeply connected.

Immune-Boosting Herbs

As the chilly winds of winter brush against our windows, many of us instinctively reach for extra layers and steaming mugs to keep warm. But fortifying our bodies against the season's bite starts from within, specifically with our immune system. Nature, in its wisdom, offers us a treasure trove of herbs that have been used for centuries to bolster health during the colder months. Integrating immune-boosting herbs into your winter regimen isn't just about staving off the common cold—it's about embracing a more resilient, vibrant self.

At the heart of these herbal remedies is *Echinacea*. Known for its potent antiviral properties, Echinacea has long been celebrated as a natural remedy for reducing the duration and severity of colds and flu. This purple coneflower isn't just a pretty addition to gardens; its roots and leaves can be turned into teas, tinctures, or supplements. By stimulating the production of white blood cells, Echinacea equips your body with an army ready to fend off winter infections.

Next, let's consider the humble *elderberry*, which has recently been thrust into the spotlight as a superfood. Rich in antioxidants, elderberries can help to lessen the severity of cold symptoms, thanks to their anthocyanins, which are known to possess immune-boosting effects. Elderberries can be transformed into delicious syrups, adding both flavour and health benefits to your winter pantry. A spoonful of elderberry syrup in warm water could become your go-to winter soother.

Astragalus, a staple in traditional Chinese medicine, is less known in the Western world but deserves attention. With its ability to enhance the body's resistance to stress and disease, astragalus root acts as a gentle yet powerful adaptogen. It works by boosting the efficiency of the immune system, making it particularly useful in preventing rather than just treating illnesses. Adding astragalus to soups and stews can be an easy and delicious way to incorporate this herb into your diet.

No discussion of immune-boosting herbs would be complete without mentioning *ginger*. This fiery root packs a punch with its anti-inflammatory and antioxidant effects. Not only does ginger help ward off sickness, but it also provides warming properties that can be especially comforting during frigid days. Add grated ginger to your tea or soup, or even enjoy it as a refreshing ginger lemon shot in the morning to invigorate your system and keep your defences up.

Another potent ally is **turmeric**, famed for its vibrant yellow hue and key active ingredient, curcumin. Curcumin exhibits strong anti-inflammatory effects, effectively aiding in reducing the inflammatory markers often associated with a weakened immune system. Combine turmeric with a bit of black pepper to increase its absorption and add a spoonful to stews, smoothies, or your morning latte for a daily immune boost.

Our exploration of immune-boosting herbs would be incomplete without acknowledging *garlic*. Often dubbed nature's antibiotic, garlic contains allicin, a compound effective against bacteria and viruses. Fresh garlic consumed regularly— either raw, roasted, or cooked— can significantly help reduce the duration of colds and bolster your body's defences.

Beyond individual herbs, combining these with other lifestyle practices amplifies their benefits. Eating a nutrient-rich diet, maintaining a healthy sleep schedule, and focusing on stress reduction are equally vital components of a strong immune system. When used intentionally and regularly, immune-boosting herbs can enhance your winter vitality and foster a sense of well-being that goes beyond mere physical health, nurturing your overall spirit.

As you incorporate these herbs into your daily regimen, it helps to remember that balance is key. Too much of a good thing can sometimes have unintended consequences, so begin with small quantities, paying attention to your body's responses and adjusting as needed. It is also wise to consult with a healthcare professional, especially if you are pregnant, nursing, or on medication, to ensure that these herbs align with your personal health needs.

Herbs like Echinacea, elderberry, astragalus, ginger, turmeric, and garlic become more than just pantry staples; they transform into companions along the winter journey. They invite you to align with nature's cycles, moving with the rhythm of the season, rather than against it. By embracing these natural allies, you're not just preserving health; you're fostering a deeper connection with the natural world and its innate capacity for healing.

This winter, let your kitchen become an apothecary, and your daily rituals a means of cultivating strength, warmth, and resilience. As you stir a pot of herbal-infused tea or prepare a meal seasoned with immune-boosting spices, know that you're not only fortifying your body but also honouring the ancient wisdom of herbal healing. Through these practices, you weave a protective cocoon around you, supporting each breath you take, each step you make, through the ebb and flow of the winter months.

Herbal Teas and Tonics

In the heart of winter, when the world is cloaked in a crisp stillness, there's something profoundly comforting about a warm cup cradled in your hands. Herbal teas and tonics aren't just about savouring warmth, but they also play an integral role in promoting winter health. Through thoughtfully chosen herbs and botanicals, these soothing infusions can bolster your immune system, lift your spirits, and offer a gentle remedy to the season's chill.

The art of creating herbal teas and tonics extends back centuries, rooted deeply in traditional practices that emphasise holistic well-being. It's fascinating to think how these concoctions were crafted in ancient kitchens, with remedies passed down through generations. Today, as we embrace these age-old traditions, we aren't just seeking health benefits but also fostering a deeper connection with nature's rhythms.

One of the simplest and most effective herbal teas is made from ginger and lemon. Ginger, renowned for its warming qualities, aids digestion and can boost circulation—perfect for those chilly days when you just can't seem to ward off the cold. Lemon, on the other hand, is packed with vitamin C and acts as a rejuvenating companion to ginger, not only enhancing the flavour but also fortifying the body's defences against winter ailments.

Another robust choice is chamomile tea, known for its calming effects. Often associated with promoting restful sleep, chamomile can also soothe the digestive tract and ease tension. A brew of chamomile flowers can transform a quiet winter evening into a restorative practice, wrapping you in a sense of calm as a gentle respite from the day's troubles.

Elderberry tonics are increasingly popular during the winter months for their reputed immune-boosting properties. Rich in antioxidants, elderberries may help reduce the duration of colds and flu. A tonic made with elderberry syrup, a splash of apple cider vinegar, and a touch of honey can be a soothing elixir for both body and soul.

For those seeking a sense of groundedness and warmth, a blend of cinnamon and clove makes for an ideal tea base. These spices bring a delightful heat and are often used in Ayurvedic practices to balance energy. Combined with black tea or an herbal rooibos base, cinnamon and clove offer a fragrant and spicy delight, infusing the home with a festive aroma that lingers as you sip.

Adaptogens, like ashwagandha and holy basil (tulsi), are increasingly embraced for their ability to help the body adapt to stress and maintain balance. Incorporating these adaptogenic herbs into your teas can support resilience, something that's especially valuable when winter's demands seem overwhelming. These herbs, often paired with spices such as cardamom, furnish a delicate brew that is both nurturing and invigorating.

Mint teas, with their bright and refreshing taste, remain timeless favourites. While they might not immediately conjure images of warmth, peppermint and spearmint are wonderful for aiding digestion and invigorating the senses. In the midst of winter, they can provide a brisk awakening that mirrors the sharpness of a frosty morning.

Crafting your own herbal blends can be both a creative and meditative process. Consider joining or hosting a winter gathering where each participant shares a favourite recipe, and together you explore new flavour combinations. This simple act of sharing can transform the ordinary into the extraordinary, fostering warmth and camaraderie that counters the solitude winter often brings.

Don't forget the beauty of citrus-infused tonics, using warming botanicals like orange peel and cardamom. Not only do these blends provide a burst of sunshine in a cup, but they also remind us of brighter days ahead. The essential oils released from citrus peels can invigorate your senses and renew your spirit—even on the greyest of days.

As we delve into the world of herbal teas and tonics, we also open our senses to the nuances of taste and aroma. Each sip can be a moment of mindfulness, an opportunity to slow down and savour life's simple pleasures. To align ourselves with nature's pace is to embrace winter with grace, learning from the stillness rather than resisting it.

The time-honoured practice of sipping herbal teas is about more than just health benefits; it's an invitation to pause, connect, and revitalise. Through every steaming mug, we're reminded that self-care is not a solitary path but a journey of interconnectedness with the world around us. Let's celebrate the winter season by inviting warmth into our bodies and hearts through the timeless ritual of tea.

Chapter 10:
Sleep and Rest for Winter Vitality

Amidst winter's tranquil embrace, sleep and rest emerge as vital pillars for sustaining vitality through the cold months. As the nights stretch longer, nature flirts with tranquillity, inviting us to synchronise our rhythms with its serene cadence. Crafting a winter sleep sanctuary becomes a soulful endeavor: enveloping your bedroom in layers of warmth, soft lighting, and soothing sounds can transform it into a refuge of calm. Explore the art of intentional napping, too— short, mindful sleep breaks that rejuvenate the spirit and sharpen mental clarity. In this season of reflection and renewal, embracing restorative sleep harnesses the innate power of rest, nurturing a resilient mind and body ready to thrive. Let the quiet of winter nights be a gentle guide into deeper rest and the rejuvenating promise it holds.

Creating a Winter Sleep Sanctuary

Winter often acts as a gentle nudge that reminds us to slow down and embrace rest. As the world outside grows colder and days become shorter, our internal rhythms naturally seek a comforting refuge. Establishing a winter sleep sanctuary isn't just a question of aesthetics; it's an embrace of well-being that nourishes our body and mind during these dormant months. By cultivating a restful environment, we allow ourselves to replenish our inner reserves and foster resilience to thrive in the cold months.

The first cornerstone in crafting your winter sleep sanctuary is choosing the right textiles. Imagine your bed adorned with layers of soft, plush blankets and warm sheets, creating a cocoon of warmth. Opt for materials like flannel or wool that hold onto heat, wrapping you in comfort. The touch of these fabrics can be transformative, their gentle embrace inviting you to drift into a restful slumber. Of course, each layer isn't just a functional choice but a sensory experience that whispers of comfort and safety.

Let's talk about the bedroom atmosphere. The air should be cool and fresh, yet balanced with warmth—about 16 to 19 degrees Celsius is often ideal for sleep. A humidifier can be your ally in combating the dryness common in heated homes, offering relief to your skin and respiratory passages. Houseplants, too, can purify the air, nurturing a sense of calm and wholeness. Plants like lavender and rosemary not only cleanse the air but their scents can lull your mind into serenity.

Lighting plays a pivotal role in defining the mood of your sanctuary. We're attuned to nature's rhythms, and exposure to the right kind of light affects our internal clocks profoundly. Consider dimming your lights as evening approaches, emulating the sunset's gentle retreat. Perhaps swap harsh overhead lights for soft, warm-toned lamps or fairy lights. Even better, use candles to draw in the deep relaxation that the flicker of their flame embodies. These small transitions can signal your body that it's time to unwind and let go.

Sound is another element that can enrich your space. Soft music, nature sounds, or white noise can gently guide you into sleep, masking any external interruptions. It's an invitation to let go of the persistent noise in your mind and find solace in the gentle ebb and flow of harmonic tones. Finding a soundscape that resonates with you can create a familiar pathway to peace, allowing anxiety to drift away.

While the practicalities are crucial, let's not forget the personal touches that make your sleep sanctuary uniquely yours. Infuse your space with items that speak to your spirit—a favourite piece of art, a family photo, or a cherished book on the bedside table. These items should evoke positive memories and a sense of belonging, enhancing the firmament of tranquillity you've built.

A technique that holds timeless value is maintaining a bedtime ritual. This isn't reserved just for children; it's a practice that can imbue your night with stability and ease. Think about a nightly routine that works for you—perhaps a warm bath laced with Epsom salts or a cup of calming chamomile tea. Spend a few moments journaling your thoughts, unburdening your mind from the day's clutter. A consistent ritual helps ease the transition from waking life to restful sleep, nurturing dreams to unfold with grace.

Harnessing the power of scent can elevate your sanctuary to new heights. Essential oils such as lavender, chamomile, and sandalwood are renowned for their calming properties. A diffuser filled with these scents can gently fill the room, their aromas weaving into your sleep narrative. These natural aromas act on a subliminal level, promoting deeper rest.

Seek mindfulness in your approach to rest. Gratitude and breathing exercises before bed can prepare your mind for the voyage ahead. This simple practice encourages a shift from the relentless pace of daily life to the stillness of the present moment, easing anxiety and paving a smoother path to sleep.

With all these elements, it's essential to remember the guideline of minimalism. Too many distractions can clutter both your space and mind. Your winter sanctuary should be a place of simplicity, where each object serves a purpose for your rest. Clutter, both mental and physical, detracts from the potential of your sleep haven to offer true replenishment.

Investing in creating a winter sleep sanctuary is an investment in oneself. It's about cultivating a comforting, serene atmosphere that aligns with the restorative nature of winter. As you nestle into your carefully curated space, you harness the quiet power of winter to renew and kindle your inner vitality, ready to face the world afresh once the sun returns. Let this sanctuary be a testament to care and compassion, the essence of your well-being during these dormant yet promising months.

Napping for Rejuvenation

Winter, with its shorter days and longer nights, naturally invites us to embrace rest and slumber more deeply than other seasons. Yet, in our modern, fast-paced lives, we often resist this call to slow down. One of the most powerful ways to harness the restorative energies of winter is through napping. While often underrated, napping has profound benefits for mental clarity, emotional balance, and physical energy, making it an essential practice for anyone seeking true winter vitality.

Understanding the art of napping begins with recognising that a nap is not a sign of laziness, but rather a strategic way to counteract the stresses and demands of daily life. Research indicates that even a short nap of 20 to 30 minutes can increase alertness and improve mood. Imagine yourself on a chilly afternoon, nestled under a warm blanket, as you drift gently into a state of rest. This simple act can rejuvenate the mind, mitigate stress, and even enhance creative problem-solving abilities.

For many, the concept of napping evokes childhood memories—those blissful midday pauses that left us feeling refreshed and ready to tackle the rest of the day. As adults, reclaiming this habit can feel like a luxury. However, prioritising a nap, especially during winter, can become a cornerstone of our self-care routine. It's about listening to our bodies' natural rhythms and allowing ourselves the grace to rest as needed.

The key to effective napping lies in timing and environment. Ideally, naps should be taken in the early to mid-afternoon when our alertness tends to dip naturally. This is the perfect window to allow ourselves a brief rest without interfering with nighttime sleep. Creating a designated nap space can also greatly enhance the experience. A quiet, dimly lit room with comfortable bedding can signal your brain that it's time to relax and recharge. Consider incorporating calming scents like lavender or chamomile through aromatherapy to deepen relaxation.

While some might worry that napping could interfere with their nighttime sleep patterns, when done properly, a nap should not replace proper nighttime rest. Instead, it serves as a supplement, offering solace during a restless day. To achieve this balance, keep naps short and sweet—aim for 20 to 30 minutes. Longer naps can lead to sleep inertia, a state of grogginess that can be counterproductive, especially if undertaken late in the day.

For those unaccustomed to napping, it might be helpful to start by setting a regular time each day to practice. Like any new habit, consistency is crucial. Over time, you'll find that your body and mind will start to adjust, and soon, napping will feel as natural as any other daily ritual. Creating a nap schedule can be a bit like creating a personal sanctuary—a time to retreat and replenish, fostering resilience and inner warmth.

In addition to the practical benefits, there's a deeply restorative aspect to napping that speaks to our spirit. Just as nature embraces a dormant phase in winter, allowing growth and renewal in the coming seasons, so too can our spirits flourish when given the proper rest. Viewing napping as a spiritual practice can enhance its benefits, turning it from a mere physical respite into an act of self-kindness and love.

To further enrich your napping practice, consider pairing it with a short pre-nap meditation. This can help clear your mind and prepare your body for restful sleep. Focus on your breath, and allow any tension to melt away with each exhale. Alternatively, listening to calming music or a guided relaxation track can create a soothing preface to your nap, enhancing the relaxation process.

As you integrate napping into your winter wellness routine, you might find surprising changes in your overall well-being. Not only can it provide a rest from the mental clutter and emotional turbulence that life often brings, but it can also reinvigorate your perspective, making everyday tasks feel more manageable and even enjoyable.

The journey toward winter vitality is personal, and napping can become a cherished part of it. By embracing this restful practice, we allow ourselves the opportunity to pause and reconnect with our inner strength. In doing so, we cultivate the resilience to face the world not as harried beings but as harmonious and integrated individuals.

In conclusion, napping offers more than just physical rest; it's a bridge to greater mental clarity and emotional equilibrium. By weaving this practice into our winter routine, we not only rejuvenate our bodies, but we also nurture our spirits, empowering us to move through the season with grace and vitality.

Chapter 11:
The Role of Light in Winter Well-being

As winter's embrace tightens, the dwindling daylight can subtly unsettle our inner equilibrium, nudging us toward introspection and, occasionally, a lingering melancholy. Yet, light—both natural and artificial—holds transformative potential in this seasonal dance. Embracing its power, we can invite renewed vitality and a profound sense of well-being into our lives. Consider the simple magic of drawing back your curtains to greet the gentle morning rays or the subtle reverie of positioning mirrors to reflect light throughout your space. Even light therapy, with its structured luminance, can become a beacon of hope, illuminating the shadows that winter casts upon our spirits. In these deliberate acts, we find not only refuge but also a path to embrace the beauty of the season, aligning our well-being with nature's rhythm. Let winter light guide the way, brightening our days and fortifying our resilience, as we bask in its gentle glow and nurture our spirits.

Light Therapy Benefits

Light, although overlooked at times, holds an intrinsic power to transform the dreary winter months into a season of potential renewal and inner joy. It's no surprise that, as the earth tilts away from the sun, some of us may feel a creeping melancholy, our spirits dimming alongside diminishing daylight. Light therapy emerges here as an unlikely hero, a beacon guiding us back to vitality and balance.

The essence of light therapy lies in its simplicity. It mirrors the sun's rays and aligns with our natural circadian rhythms, those inner clocks that tick away, synchronising our sleep-wake cycles, governing mood, and even metabolism. When daylight dwindles, some bodies cry out for what they miss: the energising touch of morning sunlight. This therapy grants that wish, flooding one's surroundings with bright, full-spectrum light that mimics natural daylight, elevating mood, boosting energy, and often easing the characteristic gloominess associated with the winter months.

Implementing light therapy can feel almost ritualistic. Begin your day by basking in its glow, ideally in those first waking hours. This practice subtly hints to your body and mind that it's time to rise and shine, chasing away the cobwebs of sleep. It's particularly vital for those who perhaps find themselves grappling with the blues as the days grow shorter, offering a gentle nudge towards happier, more vibrant days.

The benefits of light therapy stretch beyond mere mood improvement. It's a key player in mitigating symptoms of Seasonal Affective Disorder (SAD), a condition where the lack of sunlight can trigger depressive states. By integrating regular sessions of this therapy, users often note a marked decrease in anxiety and irritability, replaced by a calm focus and emotional steadiness. This palpable shift in mental clarity can encourage growth and resilience, allowing space for creativity and productivity to flourish, even amidst winter's stern grasp.

Light therapy is not just about addressing deficiencies but enhancing well-being. For some, it can improve sleep quality, aiding in the regulation of the sleep hormone melatonin. This means falling asleep more easily and staying asleep longer, nurturing your body's well-deserved rest. Imagine waking up refreshed, free from the clutches of grogginess, ready to take on the challenges of a new day, invigorated by the restorative touch of light.

Curiously, the physiological effects cascade into the physical realm as well. Regular exposure can contribute to better skin health, as light therapy has been used historically to treat specific skin conditions. While the focus remains on mental and emotional well-being, these additional benefits can act as unexpected bonuses, leaving you not just feeling good but looking it as well.

For those stepping into light therapy, it's crucial to find balance. A consistent schedule tends to yield the best results, anchoring its benefits in the ebb and flow of daily routine. It's akin to cultivating a garden; patience and regular care result in flourishing growth. The warmth of light becomes a staple, much like a cherished morning cup of tea, eagerly anticipated and thoroughly enjoyed.

Engaging with light therapy doesn't require complicated equipment or hefty investments. A modestly priced lightbox can be effective, while more adventurous souls may opt for dawn simulators, which replicate the gentle rise of the morning sun. Either way, the tools themselves can seamlessly integrate into one's sanctuary, a quiet nod to the power of light which certainly cannot be overlooked.

Ultimately, light therapy acts as a metaphor for something greater—arising from darkness and reaching into illumination. It's a tangible reminder that even in the depths of winter, each of us harbours the potential for radiance and joy. As light floods into our lives, it does more than brighten physical space; it invites us to look inward, encouraging warmth, well-being, and resilience against the cold.

While winters persist with their chill and shadows, light therapy stands as a testament to our ability to adapt and thrive. It brings to bear an understanding that, within the confluence of modern science and timeless elements, we find tools to empower our journey toward holistic health during the year's coldest span. Through this little slice of borrowed sunlight, the glow inside each one of us is already waiting to be reignited.

Enhancing Natural Light at Home

As the days grow shorter and the nights linger, the scarcity of natural light creates a unique set of challenges and opportunities for enhancing well-being during winter. This period calls for creativity and intentional design to make the most of the daylight hours we do have, transforming our living spaces into sanctuaries of light and warmth. Harnessing the power of natural light can significantly boost mood, energy levels, and mental clarity, offering a subtle yet profound impact on one's overall sense of well-being.

First, let's consider the role of windows as portals for welcoming light into our homes. Strategically placed mirrors can amplify the natural light streaming through them. By reflecting light, mirrors can effectively double the sunlight's reach, brightening areas that might otherwise remain dim. Positioning a large mirror opposite a window, or using several smaller mirrors placed at various angles, allows sunlight to dance across the room, creating an airy and uplifting ambience.

Alongside mirrors, opting for sheer or lightly coloured curtains can enhance natural light diffusion, especially during the shorter days of winter. Thick drapes might keep the cold at bay, but they can also block valuable sunlight. During daylight hours, it's beneficial to draw curtains back fully, ensuring windows are unobstructed and ready to receive every ray of sunshine.

Another way to maximise light is to consider the colour palette of your home's interior. Light colours can enhance the sense of space and reflectivity in a room. Painting walls and ceilings in shades of white, cream, or soft pastels can significantly increase the brightness of a room as these colours act as reflectors, bouncing light around and making spaces feel open and inviting. Complement these hues with metallic or glass accessories, which can further diffuse light and add a touch of elegance.

Moreover, the strategic placement of your furniture plays a critical role in promoting natural light flow. Arranging your furniture so it doesn't block windows or light paths ensures that light travels freely throughout a room. It's crucial to ensure that large pieces, like sofas or bookcases, aren't placed directly in front of windows, which could cast shadows and diminish the overall light in a space. Instead, consider placing furniture alongside windows, which can create cozy spots that receive direct sunlight, perfect for reading or relaxation.

Making small adjustments to your daily routines can also be beneficial. Aligning activities with the sunny parts of your home can offer both physical and psychological advantages. For example, moving your workspace to a sunlit area allows you to soak up natural light, potentially improving your focus and elevating your mood during productive hours. Similarly, enjoying meals in brighter spaces can make eating a more pleasant and energising experience.

Even with the best of intentions, there will be corners where natural light struggles to reach. Introducing reflective surfaces such as glass tables, metallic accents, and glossy tiles can add sparkle to these shadowed areas. These finishes can catch stray beams of light and spread them into less illuminated spaces, reducing the contrast between light and dark and crafting a balanced atmosphere.

For those eager to deepen their connection with nature, integrating indoor plants can yield surprising benefits. Not only do plants purify the air, but they also create a soothing and revitalizing environment. Positioning plants near windows draws the eye outdoors, extending the gaze beyond the glass to include the sky and changing weather patterns. This simple act of connecting with the natural world brightens both your home and your spirit.

In crafting a space that celebrates natural light, the act itself becomes a practice in mindfulness and gratitude. By noticing the way light shifts and changes throughout the day, you develop an awareness that invites appreciation for the subtle beauty of winter. Observing how sunlight slants through your home during morning, noon, and dusk invites a sense of rhythm and pace, aligning your daily activities with the natural cycles.

Finally, it's important to consider the benefits of decluttering. A tidy space allows light to move freely and dominate the room, whereas clutter can trap shadows and make a space feel cramped. Embracing minimalism, or simply committing to regular tidying sessions, can create an environment where light is maximised, offering mental clarity and a sense of peace. Streamlined spaces often evoke a more relaxed state of mind, further enhancing your emotional and psychological resilience during the winter months.

By embracing these practices with intention, you create a home that harnesses the myriad benefits of natural light during winter. Each small change builds upon another, gradually transforming your living space into a luminous haven of warmth and vitality. It's an invitation to nurture well-being by welcoming and embracing the light, even in the heart of the coldest season.

Chapter 12:
Crafting a Personal Winter Retreat

Amidst the swirling snows and twinkling frost of winter, creating a personal retreat dedicated to rest and rejuvenation can be a transformative experience. It's not about a grand getaway but rather cultivating a corner of tranquillity right within your own surroundings. Imagine designing a space that embraces you with warmth and serenity, adorned with soft textiles, calming colours, and the soft glow of ambient lighting. Within this haven, engage in activities that soothe your spirit and kindle your inner warmth—perhaps through reading, crafting, or reflective meditation. This retreat isn't confined to a physical space; it's an invitation to pause amidst winter's embrace, allowing yourself to breathe deeply and recharge. By intentionally crafting such a retreat, you're choosing to prioritise your well-being, nurturing resilience to carry through the cold months with grace and gratitude.

Designing a Relaxation Space

In the midst of winter's chill, creating a dedicated haven of relaxation can serve not only as a refuge from the cold but also as an oasis for the spirit. This space is where serenity meets sanctity, allowing you to pause and reconnect with yourself. To craft such a sanctuary, consider the atmosphere you want to foster—whether it's warmth, tranquillity, or rejuvenation—and let those feelings guide your choices.

Start by selecting a location within your home that feels right for unwinding. Perhaps it's a corner of your living room where natural light streams in, or a quieter nook in the bedroom. The most important factor is that it feels inviting and personal, a place you instinctively gravitate toward for rest and reflection.

Once the location is determined, focus on the visual elements. Soft lighting plays a crucial role in creating an inviting ambience. Consider using candles, fairy lights, or a gentle lamp with a dimmer switch, which provides the perfect glow to soothe the senses without overwhelming them. Complement this gentle illumination with a palette of warm, earthy tones or cool, calming blues and greens, reflecting the colours that naturally soothe you.

Aromatic elements can further enhance this sensory haven. Incorporate scents known for their calming properties, such as lavender, vanilla, or sandalwood. Essential oil diffusers or scented candles can infuse the air with these tranquil notes, promoting a sense of ease as soon as you enter the space.

Comfort is key in any relaxation room, so furniture and textures should be thoughtfully chosen. A plush armchair, a soft rug underfoot, or a pile of cosy blankets invites you to sink into relaxation. Consider layering different textures—perhaps a knitted throw over a velvet cushion—to add depth and tactile delight.

Adding life to your space through natural elements can be incredibly revitalising. Indoor plants not only beautify a room but also improve air quality, contributing to a refreshing environment. Choose hardy species like peace lilies or snake plants, which thrive in low light and are easy to care for.

The soundscape of your relaxation hideaway should not be overlooked. Calming music or nature sounds can mask outside noise and create an auditory cocoon, further transporting you from the hustle and bustle. Playlists with soft instrumental or ambient sounds can be curated to fit your mood or the time of day.

Personal touches make the difference between a generic room and a truly personal retreat. Consider what items make you smile—be it framed photographs, art pieces that resonate with you, or books that inspire deep thought or escapism. These tokens can act as anchors that ground your space in warmth and personality.

Your relaxation area can also be a versatile space for a variety of retreat activities. Whether it's a comfortable spot for morning meditation, a nook for journaling your thoughts, or even an area to engage in restorative yoga, ensure it's adaptable to your needs. A comfortable yoga mat or a supportive meditation cushion can easily be part of this adaptable setup.

Finally, maintaining the purity and function of your relaxation space requires mindful intention. Avoid clutter by ensuring everything in the room has a purpose. Regularly refresh the area; whether it's by adding a new flower arrangement or changing up the pillows, keeping the room dynamic will encourage you to return and recharge.

Designing a relaxation space is an act of self-love and care, offering solace during the long winter months. It serves as a sanctuary for unwinding, healing, and nurturing inner warmth—a testament to your commitment to well-being and resilience. Embrace the process, imbue it with your individuality, and let this retreat become a vital part of your daily rituals, guiding you to winter's end with inner peace and joy.

Retreat Activities

Nestled in the warmth of your carefully crafted space, a personal winter retreat invites reflection, renewal, and rejuvenation. Exploring retreat activities can deepen your connection to self-care, offering you a sanctuary to nurture your body, mind, and spirit during the colder months. These activities form the heart of your retreat, allowing you to tune into your inner world.

A personal retreat needn't follow any rigid schedule. It's about listening to your inner rhythms and needs. Some days, you might be drawn to creative endeavours, while other days may call for gentle meditation or restorative yoga. Allow your intuition to guide you, letting each day unfold naturally. Consider starting your retreat by setting an intention. What do you hope to embrace or release?

Journaling can offer a powerful outlet for processing emotions and capturing fleeting moments of clarity. Dedicate a notebook to your retreat, allowing thoughts to flow without judgement. Try a morning practice, scribbling down dreams and thoughts that arise from the night's rest. Alternatively, relive your day's experiences each evening, uncovering insights and patterns that may otherwise hide in plain sight.

Another enriching retreat activity is engaging with literature or poetry that inspires you. Choose works that resonate with your current state of mind or explore new genres that could offer fresh perspectives. Reading can be a form of meditation itself, absorbing words that transport you to new worlds or whisper profound wisdom.

Don't overlook the power of music and sound in your retreat. Curate a playlist that soothes your soul, mixing melodies that lift or calm your spirit. Music has a unique ability to resonate on an emotional level, offering comfort or catharsis when needed. Consider incorporating singing bowls or a simple chime to introduce sound healing sessions, focusing on the vibrations soothing tensions held in your body.

Creative expression is another avenue worth exploring. Whether it's painting, knitting, or playing an instrument, these activities allow your mind to wander and engage with the present. Let go of any judgement regarding the outcome. Creativity thrives in environments free from self-doubt, where the process takes precedence over the product. Use this time to rediscover joy in creation.

Meditation is central to many retreat experiences. Consider a meditative practice that incorporates movement, such as tai chi or gentle yoga. These mindful movements not only reduce stress but also enhance flexibility and balance. If stillness is more appealing, seated meditation can be equally rewarding, focusing on breath awareness or body scanning to cultivate deep relaxation.

Breathwork exercises present a powerful yet often overlooked practice to incorporate into your retreat. Techniques like alternate nostril breathing or box breathing help harmonise your body's energy, fostering clarity and balance. A few minutes each day dedicated to conscious breathing can significantly enhance your mental and physical well-being.

In addition to solitary pursuits, engaging with guided visualisations can be profoundly transformative. These visual journeys, led by audio recordings or scripts, transport you to peaceful settings or allow you to envision your future with clarity. By tapping into your imagination, guided visualisations can foster inner peace and assist in manifesting personal goals.

A retreat also provides the perfect setting to explore mindfulness practices in everyday activities. Perhaps you focus on eating, savouring each bite and texture, or engage in mindful walking, where each step becomes a meditation. Bringing mindfulness to daily actions can anchor you more deeply to the present, helping build resilience against winter's dreariness.

Craft a blend of solitude and community during your retreat. Connect with like-minded individuals who share your journey, either in person or virtually. Engaging in meaningful conversations can enrich your personal insights and reinforce shared goals through social connectivity, even amidst isolation.

A personal retreat is a chance to indulge in self-care, both inside and out. Cultivate nourishing skin and body care rituals that feel personalised and luxurious. Whether it's a soothing bath or a warm oil massage, these acts of kindness foster a sense of well-being and comfort to ease winter's harshness.

Finally, allow yourself to take breaks, relish in moments of nothingness. Unstructured rest can recalibrate your energy, giving your mind permission to wander and your body time to rejuvenate. There's no pressure to accomplish or tick off a list of activities. The true success of a retreat lies in how deeply it allows you to reconnect with yourself.

This retreat isn't a destination but a personalised journey of self-exploration and renewal. Embrace it with an open heart, and it'll offer you insight, peace, and warmth to carry throughout winter and beyond. Prioritising these retreat activities will not only illuminate the darker days but also infuse your life with newfound resilience and purpose.

Chapter 13:
Practicing Gratitude and Reflection

As we journey through the wintry landscape of self-discovery, cultivating gratitude and reflection can illuminate our path with renewed warmth and clarity. This season invites us to pause and embrace the simple joys often overshadowed by the chill. Practising gratitude daily, we unfurl the hidden gifts winter offers, like the hush of snowfall or the cozy embrace of a favourite blanket. Reflective journaling serves as a mirror to our inner world, encouraging us to explore the layers of our experiences, both joyful and challenging. By revisiting joyful memories and observing our emotional landscapes, we invite a deeper understanding and appreciation for the ebb and flow of life. In these practices, we turn inward, nurturing an inner resilience that blossoms even amidst the frost, ultimately creating a reservoir of strength and tranquility to draw from as we brave the colder months.

Daily Gratitude Practices

Practicing gratitude daily is like wrapping yourself in a protective layer of warmth and contentment, especially during the colder months. As the world outside grows frosty and the days shorter, cultivating an awareness of what we're thankful for can be a beacon of light. Becoming aware of these positives not only strengthens our resilience but also elevates our mood. Gratitude slowly builds up the capacity to find happiness in the smallest of things, and during winter, these small joys can string together to create a beautiful tapestry of well-being.

Integrating a daily gratitude practice into your routine doesn't have to be time-consuming or overwhelming. It's about weaving it naturally into the moments you already have. You might start your day by thinking of one thing you're grateful for before getting out of bed. This simple practice can set a positive tone for the rest of the day. If you're more of a night owl, reflecting on what went well before sleeping can lead to more restful and peaceful nights. Practicing gratitude at these crucial points helps anchor us in a sense of positivity, regardless of how chilly and daunting the world outside may feel.

Allocating a few moments a day to ponder on the gifts in our lives can be beautifully transformational. The key lies in making it a habit, no matter how small the act might feel. Writing down three things each day for which you are grateful can offer a tangible reminder of your blessings, even if it's as simple as the warmth of your favourite jumper or a lovely cup of tea. These written reminders can become a source of comfort on days when winter blues set in.

For some, gratitude is best experienced through the spoken word. Engaging in conversations with loved ones where you share what you're thankful for can solidify relationships and foster a deeper connection, all while strengthening your gratitude muscle. You might find that when you express gratitude to others, it encourages them to see their blessings too, creating a ripple effect of positivity and warmth that can spread through your circle of family and friends.

Incorporating gratitude into your daily practices doesn't have to stay within the confines of traditional activities. Consider combining it with an activity like meditative breathing or yoga. As you move or breathe, each inhalation and exhalation could be paired with thoughts of gratitude. "I am grateful for my body" as you stretch, "I am grateful for my breath" as you inhale deeply. This melding of movement and mindfulness can offer a profound sense of presence and appreciation, helping you to embrace the stillness of winter.

Another enriching approach is to create a gratitude jar. Each day, jot down something that makes your heart swell, fold up the note, and place it into the jar. Over the weeks, as the jar fills, you'll have a visible testament to the abundance in your life. On particularly gloomy days, dipping into this jar can bring about a gentle reminder of the light that surrounds you, inviting emotions of joy and peace even when the world outside feels starkly cold.

Visual reminders of gratitude can also enhance your practice. Keeping photographs or mementos that evoke joy and thankfulness in visible places around your home can keep gratitude at the forefront of your mind. Perhaps it's a picture of a loved one, a souvenir from a cherished trip, or even a thank-you note you've received. These items serve as daily nudges towards an appreciative state of mind, each glance allowing for a momentary pause to acknowledge the richness of life.

Incorporating gratitude into your interactions with nature during winter can also offer a new perspective. On a wintry walk, notice the glittering snow under the twilight or the unique shape of bare trees silhouetted against a winter sky. Let these moments be filled with wonder and appreciation for the beauty that exists even in the cold quietude of January. By practicing intentional gratitude in these small moments, you bolster your spirit and nurture a sense of grounding, even as the world continues to turn in its cold embrace.

Finally, remember that gratitude is a deeply personal practice. There's no need to compare your expressions of gratitude with anyone else's. What matters is finding a method that resonates with you, and allows you to foster warmth within. Let it be authentic, a small ritual you genuinely look forward to each day. Over time, as gratitude becomes second nature, it can become one of your greatest allies, lighting the way to inner warmth and resilience, one grateful moment at a time.

Reflective Journaling

As the winter months wrap us in their quiet embrace, they're a perfect time to turn inward. Our hectic routines often blind us to life's subtler nuances, but winter's slower pace allows us to pause and reflect. Reflective journaling is a powerful tool, helping us capture thoughts, emotions, and insights that might otherwise drift away like snowflakes on a breeze. It's a practice that can transform a seemingly bleak winter's day into a canvas of vibrant self-discovery and acceptance.

There's something inherently comforting about putting pen to paper. The very act of writing demands a pause—forcing the world to slow down around you. The tactile sensation of scribbling thoughts, tracing letters that form words, creates a connection between mind and body. It's a physical manifestation of the internal landscapes we often overlook. This practice, though simple, echoes with profound richness. Regular, reflective journaling invites us into the habit of actively listening to our inner voice. It gives that voice a stage upon which to declare itself, developing confidence and introspection.

But how do we begin? The initial step is to release the pressure of expectation. You don't need to write perfectly or profoundly every time. Start where you are, with what's quite simply in your heart. Let the journal be a safe container for your musings, more like a trusted confidant than a demanding critic. Today might be an exploration of gratitude for small joys, while tomorrow might unearth long-buried worries. All are welcome here, each entry a valuable thread in the tapestry of your life.

Reflective journaling isn't about dwelling in engineered eloquence. It's an exercise in authenticity. What emerges on the page might surprise you, revealing parts of yourself hidden beneath daily rigamarole or resurfacing the lessons you've learned but haven't yet recognised. Through regular practice, you'll start to see patterns that might previously have lived in the background noise of everyday life.

With each writing session, you're essentially crafting a map—an evolving guide to both who you are and who you hope to become.

Set aside a sacred space for this ritual. Perhaps you create a corner in your home nurtured by the gentle glow of candlelight or infused with calming scents from essential oils. This physical space helps cultivate mental space. Approaching reflective journaling as you would any cherished ritual imbues it with intention, transforming it from just another task into a refuge—a place to retreat and recharge, especially when the world outside feels cold and uninviting.

Once writing becomes a ritual, reflect on the graces of the season. While short days and long nights might imply scarcity, they also highlight abundance. Winter reveals how little we truly need: the warmth of a well-made cup of tea, a comforting blanket, the quiet companionship of someone dear. Journaling can be a place to express gratitude for these simple yet profound experiences. Through this practice, you start realising that an attunement to simplicity can deliver the most profound contentment.

Engage with prompts if the blank page feels daunting. Consider asking yourself questions like "What am I learning about myself this winter?" or "In what ways am I growing?" or "What am I ready to release with the melting snow?" Prompts like these can serve as gentle nudges, directing focus onto areas of your life ripe for reflection or reinvention. They offer a roadmap to the treasures that lie within your subconscious just waiting to be uncovered.

The benefits of reflective journaling are not limited to emotional well-being. There's increasing evidence suggesting its positive impact on mental and physical health. For instance, some studies show that writing about your feelings can boost immune functioning, alleviate stress, and improve sleep. It's as if by untangling your mind on the page, you bring clarity to the rest of your life, offering psychological and physiological harmony.

Winter, with its cycles of decay and renewal, reminds us that changes are a part of life. Reflective journaling helps us better navigate these transitions, embracing each phase for its lessons and opportunities. As you capture your thoughts over the months, you'll be able to look back and see your own evolution, the metamorphosis that you might have missed had you not paused to document it. It's an encouraging reminder that we are all works in progress.

Indeed, reflective journaling is profoundly personal. It's your space to dream, to vent, to plan, to grieve, and to heal. Each entry can be a mirror reflecting your soul's journey, and as you glance back through your words, you begin to appreciate the artful, albeit sometimes messy, masterpiece of your life. The practice supports a mindset of growth and a life-long commitment to inner exploration.

In conclusion, as the seasons shift from the starkness of winter to the blooming rebirth of spring, so too can you shift from introspection to action informed by insight. Let your journal be more than a collection of words—let it pulsate with life, echoing your unique voice and essence. Through reflective journaling, equipped with deeper self-understanding, you can embrace change with the gentle assurance that with each passing winter, you emerge more fully yourself.

Chapter 14:
Sustaining Motivation and Creativity

As the days draw short and the chill sets in, sustaining motivation and creativity can be a delicate dance—but it's one that holds transformative potential. Winter, often seen as a time of dormancy, actually offers a unique canvas to explore new dimensions of our own ingenuity. By tapping into the rhythm of the season, we can ignite a spark of creativity that fuels our inner fire despite the cold outside. Embrace the stillness and solitude as an invitation to cultivate new hobbies that bring joy and inspiration, like learning a musical instrument or diving into the world of intricate crafts. This is an ideal time to express yourself in unexpected ways, allowing the hush of winter to coax out hidden talents and passions you might have overlooked in busier times. As snowflakes fall and the world seems quieter, let your creative endeavours flourish, nurturing both motivation and joy with each new discovery.

Cultivating New Hobbies

Embracing new hobbies during the winter months can serve as a beacon of light through the often grey and chilly days. When the world outside seems uninviting, turning inward to discover or rekindle interests can be both rewarding and invigorating. Winter presents a unique opportunity to explore activities you might have pushed aside during busier, sun-filled months.

Long winter nights can offer the perfect backdrop for delving into creative pursuits. Whether it's painting, knitting, or writing, these activities allow for self-expression and creativity to flourish. A blank canvas or a fresh sheet of paper holds endless possibilities, inviting you to lose yourself in the process without pressure or expectation. Art in any form encourages mindfulness, offering the same calming benefits as meditation with the added joy of creation.

For those who thrive on learning, winter is an ideal time to embark on intellectual pursuits. Online courses are abundant and cover a plethora of subjects. From mastering a new language to diving deep into history or science, the options are virtually limitless. Acquiring new knowledge can boost confidence, keep the mind engaged, and brighten even the shortest of days with a sense of accomplishment and growth.

Physical hobbies shouldn't be neglected even as temperatures dip. There are myriad indoor activities that can be just as fulfilling and beneficial. Yoga, for instance, combines movement with mindfulness, strengthening both body and spirit. Indoor gardening is another rewarding pursuit. Even small spaces can accommodate a few pots or a window box. Watching plants grow and thrive despite the winter chill can be surprisingly uplifting and serves as a gentle reminder of life and vibrancy.

Crafts and DIY projects offer yet another avenue for creativity. Crafting not only results in beautiful handmade items but also reinforces problem-solving skills and boosts mood. The rhythmic nature of activities like sewing or woodworking can be meditative, helping to chase away the winter blues while adding a personal touch to your home.

Winter provides an additional excuse to take hobbies traditionally enjoyed only in solitude, and transform them into social activities. Book clubs, writing groups, or hobby clubs can create opportunities for connection without leaving the comfort of your home. These gatherings can be carried out virtually, bringing together like-minded individuals to share insights, discuss ideas, and foster camaraderie—all essential for maintaining motivation and creativity during the colder months.

If technology is a passion, winter could be the perfect time to explore it further. From coding to video editing or music production, the digital world offers boundless opportunities for creativity. Building a website, starting a blog, or producing digital art can be particularly gratifying. These hobbies not only enhance technical skills but also allow for personal expression in ways that can be shared with the wider community.

Cooking and baking can also be transformed into enjoyable and creative hobbies. Winter offers the chance to try out robust and hearty recipes, experimenting with seasonal ingredients in new ways. The act of cooking can be a therapeutic exercise, offering a sensory-rich experience that warms both body and mind. Imagine the satisfaction of crafting a homemade soup from scratch or discovering a new recipe that becomes a family favourite.

For those looking to enhance mental well-being, winter invites the exploration of solitary yet fulfilling hobbies such as puzzle-solving or chess. These activities sharpen cognitive functions and offer the rewarding challenge of strategic thinking. The quiet focus required can be deeply satisfying and provides an important counterbalance to the more frenetic pace of life.

Finally, it mustn't be forgotten that hobbies are not solely about productivity or even creativity; they're also about joy and pleasure. Pure amusement is inspiring in itself. Rediscovering a childhood pastime, such as collecting, building model kits, or gaming, can rekindle happiness and spark new ideas.

In the hustle and hard edges of everyday life, having a collection of hobbies to choose from can act as a soothing balm. Engaging in a variety of activities not only regenerates your spirit but builds resilience too. Winter, with its embrace of quiet and introspection, is an opportunity not just to embark on new creative journeys, but to uncover pathways within yourself that you may not have explored before. In these hobbies, you might find not just refuge but rejuvenation, setting the stage for seasons to come.

Creative Expression in Winter

As the cold winds whistle outside and snow begins to blanket the earth with its playful touch, winter presents a unique opportunity for creative expression. It's a season that often nudges us inward, providing a canvas—a calm, unhurried backdrop for artistic pursuits and self-discovery. With longer nights and quiet evenings, winter can be an opportune moment to dive into creative endeavours that nurture our soul and offer warmth to our thoughts.

For many, the darker days bring about a natural retreat, both physically and mentally. This introspection offers fertile soil for creativity to grow. Whether through writing, painting, music, or any form of art that speaks to you, expressing yourself during winter can foster a deep sense of fulfilment and joy. It can be as simple as picking up a pen and paper and letting your thoughts flow, unconcerned about perfection.

One way to embrace creative expression in winter is by starting a new project that aligns with the season's themes. Think of it as capturing winter's essence through art. You could try crafting your own holiday cards, creating winter-themed photo collections, or knitting a warm scarf that embodies the coziness of winter.

For writers, winter can be an inspirational muse. The stark, barren trees, the crisp air, and the muted colours offer a unique kind of beauty that invites reflection. Consider writing poetry that reflects this seasonal change, or perhaps a short story inspired by the quiet challenges and hidden joys of winter life. You might find that words come more freely as the world slows down, offering you the space to capture and articulate your thoughts in new ways.

Painting and drawing are another way to channel winter's creative energy. The subtle tones of winter landscapes, with their whites, greys, and the occasional burst of sunny yellow, can encourage artists to experiment with a different palette. Winter's stillness may drive you to explore minimalism in your work, focusing on simple lines and shapes that reflect the simplified beauty found in snow-covered scenes.

Music, too, can be a powerful form of expression during the winter months. The season's silence and serenity can be infused into the compositions, offering a soothing escape from the cold. Consider embracing the solitude of winter by composing music or learning an instrument, inviting the rhythm of the season to blend with the notes you create.

Moreover, winter offers the chance to gather with others, sharing creative pursuits in collective spaces. Whether it's a community workshop, an online painting class, or a collaborative writing group, sharing your creative space with others can bring new perspectives and techniques to your practice. It's also a great way to maintain social connections, offering warmth through shared passion even in the chill of winter.

Importantly, creativity in winter doesn't only have to revolve around traditional forms of art. Cooking can be a wonderfully creative endeavour, too. Experimenting with hearty, warming recipes using seasonal ingredients not only feeds the body but also fulfills the spirit. You could try making artful presentations of food, creating a visual feast along with an actual one.

Embrace the cosy comforts of home as inspiration for your creative projects. Look around your space for elements that inspire creativity—be it a well-worn chair by the window or a collection of cherished books. Allow these elements to be your muse, drawing on their familiarity and comfort to fuel your imagination.

Winter's transformative power lies not only in what it blankets but also in what it unveils within us. This season allows us to explore our creative potential deeply, and as we engage with our artistic side, we resist the stagnation that sometimes accompanies the starkness of winter. It's a chance to weave the contrasting threads of the season into a tapestry, one where beauty and expression come alive under the surface of white.

Revel in the process, not merely the product. By allowing yourself to create without judgement, you honour your emotions and experiences. Let creativity be your guiding light through the darker months, illuminating paths of thought and insight previously unseen.

"The only limit to your impact is your imagination and commitment," remarked a well-known voice of inspiration. This rings true, especially in winter. Art, in its myriad forms, can transcend the cold, reaching into warm corners of the heart and mind. Make creativity not just a season's hobby but a lifelong venture, growing and evolving with you as each chapter unfolds.

So, as you sit nestled in your favourite corner, a mug of steaming tea in hand, let your mind wander into realms of creativity that bring joy and warmth to your heart. The winter months may indeed be cold, but through creative expression, they can become a sanctuary, a place where the colours of the mind are as vivid as those seen on any summer day.

Chapter 15:
Guided Visualisations for Inner Peace

As the world outside wraps itself in winter's embrace, guided visualisations become an exquisite tool for nurturing inner peace. These gentle journeys of the mind invite you to explore serene landscapes and calming scenarios, crafting a sanctuary within. Picture yourself walking through a tranquil forest, the crunch of snow underfoot, or resting by a crackling fire in a cosy cabin. With each breath, tension melts away like icicles in the midday sun, leaving behind a rejuvenated spirit. Such imagery not only comforts but also bolsters resilience against the season's harsher elements. By consistently practising guided visualisations, you cultivate a reserve of calm, a quiet strength that transforms wintry solitude into an opportunity for profound inner reflection and peace.

Exploring Visualisation Techniques

The chilly embrace of winter invites us to retreat inward, encouraging a sense of tranquillity and introspection. Visualisation techniques are a powerful tool in this journey towards inner peace, offering a canvas for the mind where warmth and serenity can flourish even amidst the coldest months. As we delve into these techniques, we'll uncover how the power of the mind can transcend the physical confines of winter, fostering a nurturing internal environment that supports well-being and resilience.

At its core, visualisation is the art of harnessing the imagination to create vivid and detailed mental images. This practice, often rooted in ancient traditions, serves as a bridge between the conscious and subconscious mind. It's a way to manifest intentions, cope with stress, and cultivate a sense of calm by focusing on positive imagery. While each individual's inner landscape is unique, the process of visualisation is universally beneficial, encouraging a mental state that can significantly enhance one's quality of life during the winter season.

The versatility of visualisation makes it accessible to everyone, regardless of their experience level with meditative practices. Whether you're taking your first steps or you're a seasoned practitioner, there's a technique that can resonate with you. Some people find it easier to visualise through guided sessions, where a soothing voice leads them on a journey through picturesque settings or emotional landscapes. Others prefer personalising their practice, calling upon their own creativity to craft imagery that speaks to them individually.

A popular technique is the "Safe Haven" visualisation. This involves closing your eyes and picturing a place where you feel completely secure and at ease. It might be a real location, such as a family home or a favourite holiday spot, or an entirely fantastical setting created from scratch. The important aspect is that this place embodies peace and comfort. As you explore this haven in your mind, you can almost feel the warmth of the sun on your skin or hear the gentle lapping of the ocean waves, allowing stress and tension to melt away.

Nature-inspired visualisations can also be profoundly calming, especially during the winter months when our interaction with the outdoors might be limited. Picture yourself walking through a lush forest, the scent of pine in the air, or sitting by a crackling fire, the heat warming your face. Such imagery can evoke a sensation of warmth and connection to the earth, reminding us of the natural cycle of seasons and the promise of renewal that will come with spring.

Another powerful technique is "Visualisation for Manifestation". This involves crafting vivid images of your goals and aspirations, infusing them with as much detail as possible. By repeatedly envisioning success, joy, or fulfilment, you're essentially programming your mind to seek out paths and opportunities that align with these visions. This technique not only bolsters personal motivation but can also serve as a reminder of your purpose and desires during the more introspective winter period.

Visualisation isn't just about positive imagery; it can also be used to confront and release negative emotions. For example, you might visualise placing your stresses or worries into a balloon and watching it float away, growing smaller until it disappears from sight. This symbolic release can be incredibly freeing, allowing you to let go of what no longer serves you, creating space for peace and acceptance.

Guided visualisation sessions often come with the added benefit of an auditory component, such as soft music or nature sounds, which can deepen the relaxation experience. Consider pairing your practice with gentle, calming sounds to enhance your immersion and facilitate a deeper sense of peace. You might find that these additional sensory elements help anchor your visualisation, making it easier to return to this serene state whenever necessary.

Incorporating visualisation techniques into your daily routine can be a transformative practice, especially in winter when days are shorter and the nights longer. You might choose to begin or end your day with a brief session, allowing these mental images to set the tone for your waking hours or prepare you for restful sleep. Regular practice can help solidify these positive mental patterns, making it easier to access them in moments of stress or uncertainty.

As you explore these techniques, remember that the key is consistency and patience. Like any new skill, visualisation can take time to develop, but its rewards are boundless. Over time, you'll find your ability to conjure soothing or empowering images with ease, allowing you to draw upon this reservoir of inner strength whenever you'd like.

As we continue to embrace winter and all its gifts, visualisation offers a way to nurture and sustain our inner fire. It empowers us to create warmth and harmony within ourselves, regardless of the external chill. By mastering these techniques, we lay the foundation for a peaceful and resilient inner world, ready to thrive in any season.

Benefits of Guided Imagery

As the chill of winter envelops the landscape, we find ourselves turning inward, yearning for warmth and solace. This seasonal shift provides a perfect backdrop for cultivating inner harmony and tranquillity. One profoundly effective practice that can foster this inner peace is guided imagery. Through vivid visualization, we're able to tap into the reservoir of calm within us, transforming our mental and emotional landscape.

Guided imagery is like a journey of the mind, one where you don't need a map or even a destination. It's a practice that taps into your imagination to create a voyage filled with soothing and enlivening experiences. By picturing a tranquil beach or a serene forest, your mind and body begin to relax, mimicking the sensations of actually being in these calming environments. The power of imagery lies in its ability to engage all your senses, offering a restorative escape from life's distractions.

In the quiet hour of the day, when the world seems a little more hushed, guided imagery can bring clarity and serenity. Drifting into these visual worlds isn't just a mental exercise; it's a holistic experience influencing mind, body, and spirit. Scientific studies have shown that engaging with guided imagery can decrease stress, reduce anxiety, and even alleviate physical pain. What's remarkable is the accessibility of this practice—no special equipment or prior experience is needed. It's a gentle reminder of the power our thoughts hold.

A winter evening spent with guided imagery could mean envisioning oneself wrapped in warmth, under a sky ablaze with stars, or nestled in a cosy cabin surrounded by snowy silence. As your imagination creates these scenes, your body responds as though it's physically experiencing the scene. Your heart rate may slow, your muscles relax, and your mind finds a new clarity, unburdened by the usual chatter of daily life.

Beyond immediate relaxation, guided imagery can be a powerful tool for personal growth and change. Visualising goals and aspirations not only clarifies what they look like but also brings them into sharper focus. By regularly practising these mental rehearsals, you reinforce a positive mindset while mentally preparing for real-life scenarios. It's as though you're rehearsing for the grand performance of your life, with visualization as your trusted director.

Ancient wisdom and modern science align in appreciating the benefits of visualization. Whether you're seeking relief from a busy mind or aiming to align closer with your aspirations, guided imagery can play a pivotal role. Its effects are cumulative—the more you practice, the stronger the neural pathways associated with relaxation and positivity become. With these reinforced pathways, you're better equipped to respond to winter's stresses with grace and resilience.

The psychological benefits of guided imagery cannot be overstated. This practice helps break the cycle of negative thinking and catastrophic thoughts. When winter feels like it will never end, guided imagery allows you to mentally travel to any season or place, reminding you that your current reality is malleable and within your control. It's a gentle push against the confines of time and space, offering freedom when you need it the most.

Through guided imagery, we also nurture a deeper connection with our inner selves. It invites introspection and self-awareness, providing insights into our desires, fears, and sources of joy. For many, these sessions become more than relaxation techniques; they evolve into personal rituals of healing and discovery. As the season unfolds, these immersions offer solace and warmth, becoming intimate moments of comfort.

Imagine the impact when this practice spills into everyday life. An ability to call upon serene scenes whenever stress arises becomes a powerful ally. Whether during a challenging meeting or a long, restless night, the imagery of calm seas or tranquil forests is only a few breaths away. This mental agility becomes instrumental in negating winter's harsher moments, allowing you to remain balanced and composed.

In essence, guided imagery is about more than escaping reality. It's about reshaping it, one peaceful scene at a time. It offers a paradigm shift in coping, where instead of confronting winter's chill with resistance, you engage with it in harmony. By embracing your inner sanctuary and nourishing it with guided imagery, you're better prepared to face the winter months with renewed energy and peace.

As you incorporate guided imagery into your winter wellness routine, consider the limitless possibilities it offers. Feel free to create scenes that uniquely resonate with you, crafting environments that evoke your innermost sense of calm and strength. Guided imagery encourages imagination without boundaries, allowing you to paint your personal canvas of tranquillity. Amid the winter stillness, may you find warmth in the vibrant landscapes of your mind.

Chapter 16:
Balancing Work and Leisure in Winter

As the days grow shorter and the cool grasp of winter sets in, finding an equilibrium between work and leisure becomes essential for maintaining well-being. Winter's quiet beauty encourages us to recalibrate, urging us to align our professional demands with the pursuit of personal joy and fulfilment. The trick lies in embracing the hushed pace of the season, allowing ample room for reflection and creative exploration, alongside daily responsibilities. By weaving moments of leisure, such as indulging in a good book or savouring a warm cup of tea by the fireplace, into our routines, we foster a harmonious relationship with work that nurtures both body and spirit. Engaging in leisurely activities replenishes our energy, enhancing productivity and creativity, while reminding us that there is a time for both dedication and relaxation. This balance not only leads to a more rewarding winter experience but also anchors us in well-being that extends beyond the season's end.

Work-Life Harmony

As the chill of winter settles in, the need for a harmonious balance between work and leisure becomes almost palpable. The pace of life naturally slows during these months, offering the perfect opportunity to re-evaluate how we allocate our time and energy. Work-life harmony isn't about finding a perfect 50:50 balance between professional responsibilities and personal relaxation. Instead, it's about integrating the two in a way that enhances our overall well-being, leaving us refreshed and resilient.

In winter, daylight hours are shorter, which can often lead to a sense of urgency to get things done before night falls. This alteration in the natural rhythm can lead to increased stress and a feeling of imbalance. To counter this, it may be beneficial to adjust your working hours to align more closely with daylight, allowing yourself to bask in the sparse winter sunlight during breaks or to finish early and indulge in evening leisure activities that nourish your soul.

Imagine finishing your workday with just enough sunlight left for a brisk winter walk or an outdoor activity. These small changes can breathe life into a monotonous routine, offering mental clarity and a sense of accomplishment. Exploring flexible work arrangements, such as remote working where feasible, can significantly contribute to a sense of autonomy and balance.

Key to achieving harmony during the colder months is the establishment of firm boundaries between work and personal life. The rising trend of working from home, though beneficial, can blur these lines if not carefully managed. Designate specific areas of your home for work, thereby maintaining a clear division between professional and personal spaces. Allow these distinctions to encourage a mindset that switches naturally between focus-driven work hours and relaxation-inducing leisure time.

Our energy levels fluctuate just like the seasonal temperatures. Recognising these shifts and adapting your work-life structure can lead to more efficient productivity and deeper relaxation. Perhaps start your day with invigorating morning rituals or energising practices that set a positive tone. This groundwork can facilitate a more seamless transition into work mode, allowing for greater concentration and output.

As we adapt to our external environment, there's also an internal shift that calls for attention. Self-reflection becomes paramount, urging us to align our professional goals with personal ambitions. Use the introspective quiet of winter to realign your career objectives with personal values. Are the hours and energy you invest in work returning the joy and satisfaction you seek? Small adjustments in daily habits can start the ripple effects of change that invigorate both work and leisure experiences.

Formulating a plan that incorporates your personal passions into the weekly schedule can serve as a beacon of motivation. Engaging in activities that heighten creative expression or encourage learning can counterbalance work-related stress. For instance, consider participating in creative workshops or cultivating hobbies that bring joy and satisfaction, adding a sense of fulfilment beyond the professional realm.

Collaboration, both at work and at home, also underpins harmony. Encourage open dialogues with both colleagues and family about the challenges winter presents in maintaining balance. These conversations can foster understanding and cooperation, creating environments that support everyone's well-being. In turn, this collective effort encourages practices that benefit all, from shared outdoor exercises at lunch hours to family-facilitated relaxation sessions in the evening.

Incorporate reflective pauses in your day to assess where your energy is being expended. Mindful meditation practices can help reorient focus and encourage a grounded approach to each task. When work demands spike, these tools offer an anchor to manage stress effectively and prevent emotional burnout.

Embracing a rhythm that synchronises with winter's tempo does not mean foregoing ambition or productivity; rather, it encourages you to seek deeper connections with your intrinsic motivations. Aim for a harmonious blend of work goals with personal aspirations, recognising that both contribute to your overall vitality.

Remember, work-life harmony is a fluid endeavour. It's about feeling accomplished yet relaxed and connected rather than checked out. Use this season as a catalyst for transformation—a time to forge a path that aligns more closely with who you are and who you aspire to be, in both your work and leisure.

Ultimately, finding work-life harmony in winter requires self-awareness, adaptability, and a commitment to prioritise personal well-being alongside professional achievements. By approaching these months with a readiness to recalibrate and inspire balance, you're more likely to emerge into spring with a renewed outlook and zest for life.

Leisure Activities for Well-being

As winter unfurls its chilly embrace, finding the balance between work and leisure becomes a dance of intentional choices. Leisure activities, often underestimated, possess a profound capacity to enhance our well-being, especially in this season when daylight is sparse, and the cold seems relentless. The key is to deliberately build these moments of joy and relaxation into our lives, treating them not as luxuries but essential components of winter well-being.

Imagine curling up with a good book by the fire, the warmth radiating not just from the flames but from the stories unfolding in your hands. Reading offers a delightful escape, transporting us beyond our immediate environment without needing to step out into the cold. It allows the mind to wander through different eras, lands, and perspectives, expanding our world from the comfort of a cozy nook. Mixing up genres can add variety to this leisure activity, from fiction to non-fiction, poetry to prose, each offering its own form of escapism and enlightenment.

Knitting and crocheting have made a stylish comeback, not just as crafts but as meditative leisure activities that soothe the mind and engage the senses. The rhythm of needles clicking together can become a meditative practice, offering calm focus to the often-frenetic mind. They result in tangibles too—scarves, hats, or mittens—that give a sense of accomplishment and an added layer of warmth. Whether creating something for yourself or as a gift, these crafts propagate a deep connection—a woven bond of intention and care.

For those more inclined towards auditory experiences, music can be a powerful leisure pursuit. Listening to your favourite tunes can lift spirits, inspire creativity, and bring a sense of peace amidst life's demands. Curate a winter playlist that complements the season; include tracks that invigorate you during the workday and those that calm and settle you in the evening. Discovering new music or revisiting old favourites can become a delightful exploration of emotion and memory, weaving texture into the tapestry of your winter days.

The art of baking, with its alchemy of flour, sugar, and spices, not only warms the house with a fragrant embrace but also offers a grounding leisure pursuit. The process of measuring, mixing, and baking is an exercise in focus, creativity, and ultimately, reward. Winter is a perfect time to experiment with seasonal flavours—cinnamon, cardamom, vanilla, and nutmeg—to create treats that satisfy both the palate and the soul. Sharing these creations with family or friends can foster connection and spread joy.

Engaging in puzzles, whether they're jigsaws, crosswords, or Sudoku, can provide a fulfilling mental escape. These activities challenge the mind, pushing it to think in different ways and find solutions, all while offering a sense of achievement when completed. Puzzles are also a fantastic group activity if you're looking to spend quality time with others; they invite cooperation and communication, enhancing social bonds over a shared goal.

Another enriching activity is writing, which serves as both an outlet for self-expression and a means of reflection. Whether journaling your thoughts or composing stories and poems, writing can be a therapeutic route to understanding oneself and processing winter's unique challenges. Keeping a gratitude journal can also become a daily ritual, encouraging a positive mindset despite the season's gloom. By documenting moments of joy and thankfulness, you cultivate a habit of appreciation that can consistently refresh your spirit.

For those more physically inclined, yoga and gentle stretching exercises at home can be transformative. These activities, with their focus on breath and movement, offer a reprieve from the stress and can be adapted to suit whatever time and space you have. Whether a brief ten-minute session or a longer practice, they bring a sense of vitality and calm, countering winter's stagnation. The beauty of yoga is its accessibility, with countless online classes tailored to all levels and needs, making it a versatile option for maintaining both physical and mental health.

Painting, sketching, or engaging in any form of visual art can offer a vibrant outlet for creativity. Winter, with its stark contrasts and subtle hues, can be a profound source of inspiration. Allowing yourself to play with colours, shapes, and forms can not only improve mood but can also evoke a sense of achievement and self-expression. These expressive forms of art don't require perfection; instead, they cherish the process and the individual expression that each stroke or line represents.

Don't underestimate the power of home gardening, even in winter. Indoor plants have a magical way of refreshing spaces and boosting one's mood. Taking care of succulents, herbs, or other houseplants can become a mindful routine. Watching life unfurl in these small, vibrant bursts of green reminds us that, even in the depths of winter, nature persists. These living companions help purify the air and can be a source of calming green to counteract the often dreary winter skies.

Finally, engaging in leisure activities centred around connection—like virtual game nights or online meet-ups with friends—is crucial. These interactions nourish our social needs, vital even when in-person gatherings might be limited. Planning virtual events or casual calls can maintain those important bonds, cushioning the isolating aspects of winter.

In embracing leisure activities during winter, we tackle the season not as something to endure but as an opportunity to thrive. By weaving moments of joy and relaxation into your daily routine, you cultivate a life that balances productivity with pleasure, forming a tapestry where each moment of leisure adds richness to the fabric. This delicate balance nurtures not just the body and mind but also the spirit, affirming that winter, indeed, holds its own forms of warmth and well-being.

Chapter 17:
Music and Sound Healing

In the heart of winter, when the world is wrapped in a hushed stillness, music and sound healing can be a profound sanctuary for the soul. As the chill outside invites introspection, consider curating a playlist that resonates with warmth and serenity, harmonising with the quietude of the season. Music can uplift the spirit, accompany our meditations, and transform mundane moments into ones filled with meaning and joy. Yet, alongside melodies, silence itself holds power—a blank canvas upon which we can find clarity and peace. Embracing both sound and silence, we are reminded of their ability to hold us in balance, encouraging an inner dance of reflection and rejuvenation. Let the soothing rhythms and tranquil pauses guide you to a place of solace and healing, renewing your spirit like the gentle embrace of a fireside glow on a frosty evening.

Creating a Winter Playlist

Music has the profound ability to evoke emotions, stir memories, and craft atmospheres that can challenge the dreariness of winter. In the heart of the cold months, when the world feels quiet and introspective, curating a winter playlist becomes a powerful tool in enhancing one's mood and well-being. The right combination of songs can inspire warmth, elevate spirits, and even provide solace during chilly evenings. But how does one go about creating such a playlist that serves these lofty purposes?

When embarking on the creation of a winter playlist, it's important to first consider what you want this playlist to achieve. Are you seeking comfort during long, dark evenings, or motivation to get moving despite the cold? Perhaps you desire a tranquil backdrop for meditation or a harmonious atmosphere for gatherings with friends. The intent behind your playlist will shape the selection of tracks and ultimately determine the mood it sets.

Consider beginning your playlist with slow, soothing tunes that mirror the gentle pace of falling snow. Acoustic melodies, instrumental pieces, or songs with soft vocals can evoke a sense of calm and introspection. Artists like Norah Jones or Bon Iver often provide a gentle warmth through their music, akin to the soft glow of candlelight on a winter's night.

As you transition through the playlist, mix these softer songs with more vibrant tracks that infuse energy and warmth. Upbeat folk songs, jazz numbers, or soulful classics can lift spirits and inspire movement. Tracks from artists such as Van Morrison or Fleetwood Mac can bridge the journey from tranquillity to a more spirited atmosphere. Remember, variety, while not disrupting the playlist's continuity, is key to keeping the listener engaged.

Sound healing is another dimension to consider while curating your winter playlist. Certain frequencies and tempos have been shown to influence brain waves, enhancing relaxation or stimulating focus. Incorporating binaural beats or nature sounds—like the gentle crackle of a fireplace or the distant howl of winter winds—can provide a layer of auditory depth and healing. By tuning into these elements, you create a playlist that goes beyond entertainment and transforms into a sensory balm for the stresses that colder months may bring.

Lyrics also hold significant power. Words of hope, resilience, and warmth can echo precisely what we're trying to cultivate within ourselves during winter. Consider songs that resonate with your personal mantras of well-being. Lyrics that speak to themes of love, gratitude, and transformation can form a narrative thread throughout your playlist, serving as reminders of growth and resilience even during the most challenging winter days.

Additionally, exploring music from diverse cultures can enrich your playlist with global warmth. From the rhythmic drumming of African beats to the lilting violins of Celtic ballads, the world offers countless musical traditions that can infuse your days with new energies. This cross-cultural infusion not only enhances your musical repertoire but fosters a sense of connectedness beyond the confines of your immediate surroundings.

Creating a thematic journey within your playlist can also enhance your listening experience. Just as our days shift from morning glow to the quiet of night, your playlist can mirror these transitions. Begin with gentle and inviting morning melodies, shift to bolder tunes as the day awakens, and gradually ease back into soothing tracks as evening falls. This ebb and flow mimic the natural rhythm of life, grounding us amidst winter's more turbulent moods.

Once your playlist is crafted, it can become a valuable companion throughout the season. Whether playing softly in the background during a quiet afternoon at home or serving as a catalyst for movement during a morning workout, the playlist becomes a fixture of your winter routine. It welcomes shared moments with others or provides solace during solitary reflection, thus becoming intertwined with your winter experience.

Do not hesitate to refine and revisit your playlist as the season progresses. Add new songs that resonate with the passing of weeks, remove those that no longer align with your emotional landscape. Embrace the playlist as a living entity that evolves with you, much as the winter landscape outside your window shifts and changes each day.

In creating a winter playlist, you are essentially crafting a soundtrack for your winter self-care journey. It is an invitation to explore your own emotional landscape through the transformative power of music. As you cultivate warmth and resilience through each song choice, you are, in essence, nurturing the heart and soul, ensuring they remain vibrant even as the days grow shorter and the nights colder.

Thus, allow yourself the freedom to explore and experiment musically, finding those sounds that genuinely warm your spirit. Whether it is the soulful whisper of a violin or the invigorating beat of a drum, let each note guide you toward an inner refuge where winter's chill cannot intrude.

The Power of Silence

Amid the symphony of life, the profound impact of silence is often overlooked. In the context of music and sound healing, silence isn't merely the absence of sound; it represents a powerful, intentional pause that brings balance to our auditory experiences. When embraced, these moments of quiet can foster a deeper connection to ourselves and the world around us.

Silence allows us to listen inwardly, engaging with our thoughts and emotions without distraction. In the winter months, when the world is naturally quieter, this silence becomes a canvas for self-discovery and healing. It invites a serene introspection that can be both comforting and enlightening. Just as nature hibernates to replenish its vitality, we too can retreat into silence to nurture our inner warmth and resilience.

Sound therapists often incorporate silence strategically between tones and rhythms. These pauses aren't random; they're calculated spaces, providing a neutral ground amidst complex harmonics. In this silence, the body can process the healing properties of sound vibrations. The quiet holds a mirror to our inner turmoil and tranquillity, offering a chance to observe without altering the state of our minds.

Scientific studies highlight the impact of silence on the brain. A study published in the journal *Heart* found that silence can be more relaxing than listening to music, with just two minutes of silence proving to have a stronger calming effect than noting else. Silence lowers blood pressure, slows heart rates, and encourages an overall decrease in stress levels by altering the flow of adrenaline in the body.

Incorporating silence into everyday life doesn't have to be complicated. You can start by creating small pockets of silent time in your daily routine. These could be moments spent enjoying a cup of tea without distractions or sitting quietly before starting your day. Engage in mindful walks where you consciously disconnect from technological noise. Allow your surroundings to speak subtly to you through the rustle of leaves or the distant hoot of an owl.

The quiet can be intimidating at first. Many of us are unaccustomed to the absence of noise, equating it with loneliness or disquietude. Yet, as we embrace silence, we begin to understand its language. It's in this understanding that we discover its power – a power not to isolate but to connect more deeply with ourselves and our surroundings.

Silence also enriches our communication. In relationships, it's in those quiet moments shared with others that deeper connections are often found. During conversations, allowing silence to fill the space can offer clarity and depth that words sometimes fail to achieve. It's a subtle reminder that listening can be as powerful as speaking.

Moreover, the practice of meditation is deeply intertwined with embracing silence. It employs quietness as a tool for focusing the mind and achieving a state of calmness and balance. As part of a winter self-care routine, meditative silence can help anchor us amidst external chaos, enhancing our ability to cope with the seasonal challenges that winter brings.

For those sceptical about integrating silence into their healing practices, start with guided meditations that use silence deliberately between spoken guidance. As one becomes comfortable, these spaces of silence can be expanded, allowing the participant to explore their depths of consciousness undisturbed by external inputs.

Winter provides a unique opportunity to harness the power of silence. The shortened days and longer nights naturally promote introspection and contemplation. This seasonal quietude can serve as a haven from the relentless noise of our busier months, inviting you to pause and reflect on the year past and the months ahead.

With each practice session where silence is embraced, you may find yourself emerging refreshed, with a profound sense of peace and an enriched capacity for empathy and understanding. Thus, silence becomes not a void but a vital component of our well-being journey, especially amidst the winter cold.

As you embark on this venture into the uncharted realm of silence, remember that this is not an instant process but a gradual unfolding. Each moment of silence is a step closer to a steadier, more resilient version of yourself, equipped to face the challenges winter eagerly presents. Relish these moments; they are as fleeting as a snowflake's delicate landing, as eternal as the world's whispered secrets.

Chapter 18:
Winter Travel and Adventure

In the throes of winter, a world of travel and adventure awaits those who seek a different kind of warmth—a vivid tapestry of experiences that ignite the spirit and embrace the season's unique charm. From the vibrant Northern Lights dancing across Arctic skies to serene escapes in snow-laden forests, winter's canvas unfurls a myriad of destinations tailored for both thrill-seekers and solace-seekers alike. This season invites us to embark on journeys that challenge our boundaries, both physical and emotional, as we glide down pristine slopes or meander through cobblestone streets frosted in delicate white. The key to unlocking winter's potential lies in preparation; layering up in cosy attire and packing essentials to ensure comfort and safety. Whether you're carving paths on icy trails or savouring a moment of stillness in a rustic cabin, winter travel becomes an adventure of self-discovery and resilience. Engaging with winter in this way not only enriches our understanding of its beauty but also fortifies our inner strength in navigating the chilly climes of both nature and life.

Destinations for Winter Travel

As we venture into the heart of winter, the season invites us to explore destinations that not only boast stunning landscapes but also offer unique experiences for rejuvenation and adventure. Travelling during the winter months provides a chance to break away from the routine, to re-discover awe in snow-kissed vistas, and to embrace the thrill of exploring the world in its frosted glory. Whether one seeks serene isolation or vibrant festivities, the right winter destination can become a sanctuary that warms the heart and stirs the soul.

For those seeking tranquillity and a slower pace of life, the Nordic countries offer a mesmerising escape. Imagine retreating into the vast stillness of Finnish Lapland, where you can witness the mesmerising dance of the Northern Lights from the warmth of a glass igloo. The sheer scale of the arctic wilderness invites introspection, allowing the mind to quieten as reindeer softly tread through snow-covered landscapes. Here, the gentle embrace of a wooden cabin, complete with a crackling fire and a hot sauna, provides the perfect backdrop for reflection and relaxation.

In stark contrast, the Austrian Alps beckon those who crave high-energy escapades. Known for their pristine slopes, they offer some of the best skiing experiences in the world. The challenging terrains promise an exhilarating affair for adventure enthusiasts. But it's not all about adrenaline; the alpine villages, with their fairy-tale charm, present an opportunity to indulge in the warmth of local hospitality. Cosy cafes entice with steaming mugs of hot chocolate, while the après-ski culture offers both camaraderie and comfort.

Crossing over to the lush landscapes of New Zealand, the Southern Hemisphere promises a summer twist to your winter journey. The vibrant cities are complemented by breathtaking nature, presenting diverse activities from hiking through lush rainforests to lounging on sun-drenched beaches. The harmonious blend of adventure and relaxation makes this a refreshing destination for those looking to escape the northern chill while still connecting deeply with the natural world.

However, if warmth and cultural immersion are what you seek, the vibrant streets of Morocco might be your calling. Marrakech, with its bustling markets and rich tapestries of life, offers an exotic escape. As the winter sun bathes the streets in golden light, the lively souks brim with the aromas of spices and freshly brewed mint tea. Here, amidst the labyrinthine alleyways and the calls of merchants, there's a unique opportunity to reconnect with the richness of human connections and the simplicity of life's pleasures.

For those drawn to the transformative power of nature, Yosemite National Park in California is a winter wonderland. The iconic landscape is transformed under a blanket of snow, offering a serene retreat for reflection and inspiration. With trails that meander through silent forests and around frosted lakes, it's easy to find moments of solitude. Stargazing in the clear, crisp night sky underscores nature's immense beauty, providing both a humbling and uplifting experience.

Meanwhile, Japan's Hokkaido presents a cultural tapestry interwoven with natural splendour. Famed for its powdery snow, it draws winter sports enthusiasts from all corners of the globe. Beyond the slopes, the region's hot springs, or onsen, offer a balmy reprieve from the cold, blending the therapeutic benefits of geothermal waters with breathtaking mountain views. This, paired with the traditional elements of Japanese culture, fosters a deep sense of harmony and well-being.

Travelling to warmer climes, the Mediterranean islands offer an idyllic winter retreat. Cyprus, bathed in winter sunshine, combines historical intrigue with restful beaches. The sea remains inviting, and the ancient ruins tell stories of civilisations past, allowing for gentle exploration. The mild temperatures and rich cultural heritage provide a perfect mix for those wishing to keep winter's chill at bay while nurturing their spirit of curiosity.

Finally, for those inspired to venture further, the rugged landscapes of Patagonia, straddling the borders of Chile and Argentina, present unconquered beauty. Under the expansive Patagonian skies, ice fields, towering peaks, and deep fjords evoke a sense of awe. The profound tranquillity here invites contemplation, as the raw, untouched wilderness serves to remind us of nature's enduring majesty.

In choosing a destination for winter travel, consider not just the place but the experience you wish to cultivate. Do you seek solitude or shared joy? Adventure or repose? Every journey can echo with self-discovery and reflection, enticing you to step out of your comfort zone, embrace the newness of winter's embrace, and return home with stories woven into the fabric of your being. Each destination, in its distinct way, offers more than a break from the routine—it offers a chance to ignite your inner fire, to connect more deeply with yourself and the world around you.

Preparing for Winter Adventures

As we delve into the heart of winter, the call to adventure is unmistakably crisp and invigorating. The allure of snow-clad mountains, the enchantment of frost-kissed forests, and the promise of unique experiences beckon us to explore beyond the comfort of our homes. But before embarking on these winter ventures, a mindful approach to preparation can transform these excursions from taxing trials to joyous journeys.

There's something inherently magical about winter travel. It's a time to witness the world anew, cloaked in a serene white canvas that invites you to imprint your own adventures upon it. Whether you're planning a trek through snowy landscapes, skiing down powdery slopes, or simply exploring winter markets, the first step lies in understanding the specific demands of the season. After all, winter adventures require not just enthusiasm but also a thoughtful readiness to embrace the elements.

Packing for a winter getaway requires a strategic mindset. Layering is your best friend—think breathable base layers to wick moisture away, insulating middle layers for warmth, and windproof outer layers to shield you from the elements. Invest in high-quality gear like waterproof boots, gloves, and a sturdy hat, which are indispensable in keeping you comfortable and protected. Remember, when you're warm and dry, you're more likely to relish every moment of your journey.

As you map out your itinerary, safety should be top of mind. Research the weather conditions of your chosen destination, and be prepared for sudden changes. Winter landscapes can be unpredictable; it's crucial to stay informed and flexible. Equip yourself with essential tools such as maps, a compass, and a charged mobile device, ensuring you have a means to stay on course and connected. Familiarising yourself with emergency procedures can also add an extra layer of security.

One can't overlook the necessity of physical preparation. Winter sports and activities can be demanding, so maintaining a fitness routine that builds stamina, strength, and flexibility is advantageous. This doesn't mean you need to be an athlete but incorporating exercises that target your core, legs, and endurance can make your winter escapades more enjoyable and less strenuous.

Nurturing mental resilience is equally important. The challenges of winter adventuring, from long treks to navigating inclement weather, require not only physical readiness but also mental fortitude. Practising mindfulness and meditation can bolster your resolve, helping you stay present and positive even when conditions are less than favourable. Having a positive mindset can turn daunting moments into opportunities for growth and self-discovery.

Fuel your body with the right nutrients to sustain your energy levels during winter adventures. Adequate hydration is often overlooked in cold climates, yet it remains critical. Warm beverages such as herbal teas or infused hot water can keep you hydrated and warm. Also, pack nutrient-dense snacks like nuts, dried fruits, and energy bars that provide sustained energy without weighing you down.

As you prepare to face the wintry outdoors, consider the balance between adventure and self-care. While pushing your limits can be rewarding, it's also essential to listen to your body and know when to rest. Building in downtime can rejuvenate your spirit and make your experiences more enriching. Acknowledging when to pause and soak in your surroundings can turn an adventure into a soulful journey.

This season offers a distinctive perspective to connect with the natural world and yourself. As you trek through silent woods or stand atop a snowy peak, allow yourself a moment of reflection. Breathe in the crisp air and let it fill you with vitality and a sense of wonder. Winter adventures are not just about the destinations we reach but also about the inner journeys we navigate along the way.

Your winter adventures await, brimming with possibilities and untold stories. By adopting a well-rounded approach that encapsulates preparation, resilience, and openness to discovery, you transform the cold into a canvas of serenity and adventure. Embrace this season's opportunities, and let the adventure unfold as a testament to your spirit's warmth and resilience.

Chapter 19:
Spiritual Practices for Inner Fire

Winter's chill can make the spirit feel a bit weary, yet it's a perfect time to ignite an inner fire through spiritual practices. Embracing the stillness of the season, we can delve into rituals that restore and renew. This chapter invites us to explore the deep connection between winter and spirituality, where the cold surface can give way to profound warmth within. Practice mindfulness in the soft glow of candlelit quietness; each flicker becomes a gentle teacher of presence. Meditative breathing, akin to the rhythm of falling snow, allows for a release of tension and a welcoming of peace. Engaging in simple, heartfelt rituals can transform darkness into a season of introspection and soul nourishment. Whether through meditative walking in frosted landscapes or by sharing gratitude in moments alone, winter offers a unique space for spiritual reflection and growth, fostering a resilience that burns brightly, even against the backdrop of the longest nights.

Exploring Winter Spirituality

As the winter months embrace us with their crisp chill and long evenings, they also offer a unique opportunity to venture inward and explore the rich tapestry of winter spirituality. It's a season that invites us to pause, to connect with deeper meanings, and to seek tranquility in the quietude. Just as nature retreats to rejuvenate and prepare for new life, so too can we use this time to cultivate our inner fire through spiritual practices that might otherwise be overshadowed by the hustle of warmer months.

Winter spirituality isn't about distancing ourselves from the external world; it's about nurturing a sense of inner warmth and clarity. This is the time to delve into practices that resonate with the themes of stillness and reflection. You might find inspiration in the dark, starry skies that echo the vastness of our universe or in the quiet rustle of a snowy evening, reminding us of the beauty of silence and stillness.

One powerful way to explore winter spirituality is through meditation and breathing practices specifically tailored for this season. The act of sitting quietly, allowing the mind to settle and the breath to deepen, can be particularly grounding. These practices can foster a sense of warmth and peace within, helping you navigate the darker days with a gentle grace. Visualising a warm, golden light enveloping the body can be a simple yet effective technique to cultivate inner warmth and to activate your inner fire.

Incorporating rituals into your daily routine can also enhance your connection with winter spirituality. Consider lighting candles at dusk to symbolise the light within amidst the darkness. This simple action can transform a mundane activity into a sacred moment of reflection. Another practice is creating an altar or a sacred space at home. Adorning it with objects that hold personal meaning or evoke a sense of peace can serve as a daily reminder of your spiritual intentions.

Exploring winter spirituality isn't confined to solitary practices. Engaging with community and shared rituals can offer warmth and a deeper sense of connection. Gathering with others for a winter solstice celebration or joining a community meditation group can reinforce the shared nature of these spiritual explorations. The energy generated in group settings can enhance your personal practice and offer new perspectives and inspiration.

Embracing nature during winter is another pathway to deepen your spiritual connection. Even in the cold, nature offers its own kind of warmth and wisdom. Winter landscapes can whisper truths about resilience and the cyclical nature of life. A simple walk in the woods, observing the interplay of light and shadow, can become a meditative experience, encouraging reflections on personal growth and transformation.

It's also a season for storytelling and reflection, drawing inspiration from ancient myths and legends that celebrate the transformative power of winter. Many cultures have rich oral traditions that speak to winter's magic—stories that symbolise rebirth and renewal. These tales, often told by the fireside, can kindle our inner spirit and remind us of the cyclical nature of life.

In exploring winter spirituality, remember that it's a deeply personal journey. There are no rigid rules or expectations—what resonates with one person may not with another. You might find solace in journaling your thoughts and spiritual insights, capturing moments of clarity or inspiration as they arise. Reflective journaling can serve as a companion, providing insight into your spiritual progress through the colder months.

Music, too, plays a role in nurturing our spiritual self during winter. Creating a playlist of soothing, uplifting music can enhance your meditation or reflective practices. Music has the power to evoke deep emotions and can transform a simple moment into a spiritual experience. This auditory sanctuary can be a refuge during the winter months, lending an aural warmth to balance the outer cold.

Ultimately, the exploration of winter spirituality is a journey toward inner warmth, resilience, and balance. It's about honouring the season's invitation to slow down and listen to the whispers of your soul. By embracing these practices, we can emerge from winter's cocoon more illuminated and prepared for the renewal of spring, having fostered a deeper connection with ourselves and the world around us.

Rituals for Renewal

Winter's embrace offers a unique canvas for introspection and renewal. In the heart of cold days and long nights, we find an opportunity to strip away the extraneous and focus on what truly fuels our spirit. Rituals for renewal are sacred practices that connect us with our inner fire, reigniting passion and resilience amidst the frosty embrace of winter. These rituals are not just acts but become the pulse of our inner transformation, allowing us to emerge more vibrant and in tune with ourselves.

Initiating a ritual for renewal starts with intentionality. Imagine each breath as an invitation to release old patterns and welcome fresh beginnings. Set a time, a place, and a purpose. Let it be your sanctuary where time pauses, leaving room for your spirit to expand. Incorporate ambient sounds—such as gentle winds and rustling leaves—by playing nature soundtracks to create an auditory canvas that mirrors the season's serenity.

Lighting a candle can serve as a pivotal moment of transition. The flickering flame symbolizes the warmth of hope and the light within. As you light the candle, focus on the intention you wish to set. This simple act can be immensely powerful, drawing parallels between the act of lighting an external flame and igniting your own inner fire. Candles with natural scents like cedarwood, pine, or cinnamon can also infuse the air with a sense of calmness, further weaving the fabric of your winter sanctuary.

Rituals often involve elements of nature, drawing from the earth's own transformative stages. Consider integrating symbolic elements that resonate with the season. Pine cones, representing endurance and potential new life, can be gathered to form a central piece in your ritual space. An evergreen wreath or branches remind you of nature's resilience, encouraging you to draw parallels with your own capacity to endure and flourish through adversity.

Incorporate meditation or silent reflection into these rituals. Just a few moments of stillness each day can serve as a mental and emotional reset. During this time, focus on your breath, grounding yourself in the present moment. Reflect on the nourishment winter brings, not only to the environment but also to your soul. This practice can help heighten your awareness of the internal rhythms aligning with the season's energies.

Writing can also be a profound component of a renewal ritual. Keep a winter journal where you can jot down thoughts, feelings, or aspirations. Record observations about changes in your internal landscape, or sketch out imagery that speaks to your journey. Journaling is not just about writing; it's an invitation for deep reflection, a chance to pour out your heart onto paper, making room for new experiences and emotions to flourish.

Visualisation adds another layer to these rituals, invoking the power of imagination to inspire and rejuvenate. Picture the turning of the seasons within you. Envision the thawing ice and budding potential lying dormant beneath the surface. Let this imagery motivate you, providing a mental map for transformation and growth. The use of vision boards can be a tangible representation of these visualisations, offering a daily reminder of your intentions and the spirit of renewal.

Engage in movement as part of your renewal ritual. Whether it's yoga, tai chi, or a gentle stretching routine, movement invigorates the body and aligns with the transformative energy of winter. Guided by deep, rhythmic breathing, each movement becomes a dance with your inner self, loosening stagnation and inviting vitality. Choose movements that resonate with you, fostering a connection between mind, body, and spirit.

Integrate music into your rituals. Sounds can lift our spirits and transport us emotionally to where words alone might fail. Curate a playlist that resonates with the themes of renewal, invoking a sense of wonder and hope. Allow the melodies and harmonies to flow through you, each note a thread weaving its way through the tapestry of your spirit.

Communal rituals can foster a shared sense of renewal. Gather with friends or family to create a shared renewal space. These gatherings can be simple yet meaningful. Sharing stories, intentions, or even simple breaths of gratitude can magnify the energy and intention of renewal, turning each participant into a beacon of warmth and support for one another.

As we undertake these rituals, remember that renewal is not about erasing the past but about honouring it while shaping the future. Each ritual is a reminder that, although winter may cloak the world in silence, beneath it all lies a symphony of potential. With every practice that nurtures our inner world, we stitch together the fabric of our being—moving towards the light that breaks at winter's end.

Let these rituals be a guide, not a prescription, to your personal journey of renewal. Embrace the winter as a time to gently rekindle the flames of your spirit, trusting that the warmth you cultivate within will illuminate your path long after the snows have melted.

Chapter 20:
Coping with Seasonal Affective Disorder (SAD)

As the winter months unfurl their long nights and muted days, many individuals find themselves grappling with the insidious embrace of Seasonal Affective Disorder (SAD). This seasonal challenge, rooted in a complex interplay of reduced sunlight and disrupted internal rhythms, can cast a formidable shadow over our mental landscapes. However, understanding SAD becomes the first step towards empowerment. Embracing a tapestry of strategies can illuminate even the darkest days. Incorporating light therapy not only mimics sunshine but also rejuvenates the spirit, offering a daily ritual of hope. Engaging in physical activities, even in the colder months, helps release mood-enhancing endorphins with each brisk walk. Meanwhile, nourishing the soul with comforting meals abundant in omega-rich foods and vitamin D supplements fortifies our emotional resilience. As we weave these practices into our daily routine, let the harmony of soothing routines and creative pursuits guide us back to balance and well-being, reminding us that even winter's chill bears the possibility of warmth and renewal.

Understanding SAD

Seasonal Affective Disorder (SAD) is a complex condition that affects many individuals as the days grow shorter and the nights stretch longer during winter. While it's often colloquially referred to as the "winter blues", SAD is a recognised form of depression that typically occurs at the same time each year. Understanding SAD begins with recognising its multifaceted nature, deeply rooted in the interplay between our body's biological functions and the environment.

For some, the onset of SAD might feel gradual, like a slow encroachment of darkness. For others, it's as abrupt as the plunge in temperatures. One of the most profound influences on SAD is the reduction in daylight. We are creatures of light, with our internal clocks, or circadian rhythms, synchronised to the sun. When daylight diminishes, it disrupts this natural rhythm, leading to changes in mood and behaviour.

This disruption can have cascading effects. Reduced sunlight can lead to lower levels of serotonin, a neurotransmitter crucial for mood balance. Concurrently, the change in daylight affects melatonin levels, a hormone that helps regulate sleep. Heightened melatonin levels can make us feel lethargic and sluggish. With these biological shifts, the mind and body may struggle to maintain their usual levels of energy and motivation.

Symptoms of SAD go beyond mere sadness. Individuals may experience persistent low moods, a lack of interest in activities, changes in appetite or weight, and sleep disturbances. Additionally, these symptoms can be accompanied by irritability, feelings of despair, and difficulties in concentrating. Such outcomes can seem overwhelming and bewildering, yet they are responses to intricate internal processes rather than signs of personal weakness.

It's essential to distinguish SAD from typical winter dissatisfaction. While many people might feel less energetic during colder months, SAD is characterised by more severe symptoms that can interfere significantly with daily life. Recognising the line between general winter blues and SAD is crucial for seeking the appropriate help and interventions. Diagnosis often involves a combination of self-assessment and professional consultation, ensuring that individuals receive the support they need.

Biology plays a considerable role, but genetic predisposition and personal history contribute too. Those with a family history of depression or SAD are more likely to experience it. Additionally, women's likelihood of receiving a SAD diagnosis is markedly higher than men's, although the reasons remain an area of ongoing study.

What also makes SAD a unique challenge is its predictability. While the anticipation of SAD's return may feel daunting, this predictability, paradoxically, offers a chance for preparation. Understanding its cyclical nature means that sufferers can prepare strategies and interventions ahead of time, reducing its impact.

This understanding invites a compassionate perspective towards oneself. By acknowledging and accepting the condition, one can take constructive steps towards management and healing. Rather than shying away from recognising SAD as a medical condition, it's empowering to view understanding as the first step in harnessing tools for betterment.

Managing SAD often involves a multi-pronged approach. Medical treatments such as light therapy, which involves exposure to bright artificial light, have shown efficacy in alleviating symptoms by simulating the sunlight the body craves. In some cases, cognitive behavioural therapy (CBT) is recommended to reshape the negative thought patterns that accompany SAD. Antidepressant medications may also be prescribed for more severe cases.

While professional help is invaluable, personal lifestyle adjustments can significantly aid those living with SAD. Regular exercise, although challenging in colder months, has proven benefits for mental health by boosting serotonin levels and improving sleep. Even gentle activities like yoga or dance can make a difference.

Moreover, maintaining a balanced diet rich in omega-3 fatty acids can support brain health and mitigate mood fluctuations. Foods such as salmon, flaxseeds, and walnuts can be small yet impactful additions to one's diet. The act of cooking and sharing meals can also enhance one's emotional state, providing warmth and connection during colder months.

Understanding SAD encompasses both knowledge of its effects and a toolkit for coping. It's a journey of familiarising oneself with how seasonal changes affect the psyche and setting up defences to promote well-being. When one steps back to view winter as a time for inner cultivation rather than a prolonged period of survival, the challenge of SAD becomes an opportunity for resilience and growth.

Embracing winter's lessons means tuning into one's inner experience and reaching out for support when needed. By crafting a supportive environment and leaning on available resources, navigating the harshest months becomes more feasible. Accepting that it's okay to need a little more light and care allows individuals to build a fulfilling winter, despite SAD's challenges.

In conclusion, understanding SAD is recognising the deep influence of the seasonal cycle on the human mind and body. It's about honouring this connection while adopting techniques that foster light and warmth within. With awareness, preparation, and compassion, it's possible not just to survive but to thrive during the winter months, turning what might have been a daunting ordeal into a period of transformation and self-care.

Strategies for Managing Symptoms

Facing the winter months with Seasonal Affective Disorder (SAD) can feel like a daunting task. However, implementing effective strategies to manage symptoms can transform this challenging period into an opportunity for growth and self-discovery. While it's perfectly natural to feel apprehensive as the days grow shorter and the nights longer, it's also an invitation to develop a toolkit that fosters resilience and well-being. By focusing on specific strategies, you can find your rhythm amidst the winter's embrace.

One of the primary approaches for managing SAD is to remain in tune with natural light as much as possible. Light therapy, a tool frequently recommended by experts, involves using a lightbox that mimics natural sunlight, considerably brightening the room and your mood. It is most effective when used consistently, ideally in the early morning, to help regulate your body's internal clock. In tandem with light therapy, seeking moments of outdoor exposure to daylight can be remarkably beneficial, even on overcast days. While it may be tempting to linger indoors, a brief walk during the daylight hours can uplift your spirit and invigorate your senses.

Establishing routine can be a cornerstone for managing symptoms of SAD. A structured daily schedule not only promotes stability but also offers a comforting rhythm during an otherwise uncertain time. Integrating activities that bring joy, whether it's practicing yoga, engaging in creative arts, or spending time in nature, plays a vital role in maintaining mental wellness. As winter tries to confine you, creating an internal landscape of warmth and joy combats the external cold, building a resilient spirit ready to face whatever comes.

Another important aspect is maintaining social connections. The instinct to isolate during the winter months can intensify feelings of loneliness and sadness. Counteracting this requires intentional effort to reach out and connect with loved ones, whether through a cosy gathering over a warm meal or a simple phone call. Regular interaction can help uplift your mood, providing reassurance and support, reminding you that you are not alone as you navigate the complexities of SAD.

In addition to these practices, a balanced diet can support overall mental health. Winter often brings cravings for heavier, comfort foods, but ensuring that your diet remains rich in essential nutrients while satisfying those cravings can help stave off mood dips. Foods high in omega-3 fatty acids, like salmon and walnuts, alongside those rich in vitamin D, can be particularly beneficial. Taking time to prepare and savour meals can also become a moment of mindfulness, diverting focus away from worries and towards nourishment and gratitude.

Exercise is another powerful ally. Physical activity releases endorphins, which are natural mood lifters, helping counteract the lethargy and apathy that often accompany SAD. Even light to moderate exercise, such as walking, stretching, or dancing in your living room, can significantly improve how you feel. It's about moving your body in ways that feel joyous and accessible, reinforcing that energy begets energy.

Meditation and mindfulness exercises hold potential for solace and resilience. These practices teach you to anchor in the present moment, fostering an awareness that helps manage anxious thoughts and feelings of sadness. Set aside time each day for mindful breathing or a brief meditation session, creating a sanctuary for the mind amidst the noise of daily life. This pause can become a sacred ritual, safeguarding your mental health, and creating a buffer against seasonal challenges.

A minor but impactful change can include enhancing your living space. Create a sanctuary that comforts and inspires, using warm lighting, soft blankets, and uplifting scents. Colors and textures can influence mood more than you might think, and a nurturing environment can make a significant difference in how the winter months are experienced.

Sometimes, combating SAD might require professional support. Therapy, particularly cognitive behavioural therapy (CBT), can provide valuable insights and techniques for managing symptoms.

Engaging with a therapist offers a safe space to explore deeper emotional patterns, encouraging personal growth. While SAD can feel isolating, tapping into professional resources can remind you that help is always within reach, opening doors to new ways of understanding and healing.

Incorporating sound and music therapy can also play a role in managing symptoms. Creating a playlist filled with empowering and soothing tunes can help shift and elevate your mood. Moreover, embracing silence as a form of healing, removing external noise to listen inward, can invite a serene peace that allows you to centre yourself amidst winter's demands.

Another often overlooked strategy is the power of regular sleep patterns. Aim for consistent bed and wake times every day to help regulate your internal clock, promoting a sense of balance and stability in your life. Quality sleep is deeply interconnected with your emotional health, and establishing healthy sleep hygiene practices can provide a solid foundation for managing the challenges posed by SAD.

Finally, the power of reflection shouldn't be underestimated. Regular journaling fosters awareness and creates a space for reflection, allowing you to track your emotional fluctuations and celebrate progress. This practice encourages gratitude and acknowledges the quiet triumphs that come with each passing day, cultivating a sense of accomplishment and inner warmth.

While Seasonal Affective Disorder presents real challenges, it also offers opportunities for greater self-understanding and resilience. By embracing a combination of these strategies, you empower yourself to not only endure the winter months but thrive within them, tapping into a wellspring of inner strength and warmth that goes beyond the seasonal chill.

Chapter 21:
Nutrition for Energy and Warmth

As winter's chill wraps around us, nourishing our bodies with the right nutrients can be a beacon of warmth and vitality. In this season, food isn't merely sustenance; it's a source of energy, comfort, and resilience. Embrace warming foods—root vegetables, pulses, spices—each offering a unique blend of nourishment deeply attuned to the season's rhythm. They not only fuel our physical needs but also kindle an inner glow that sustains our emotional and mental well-being. By crafting balanced winter meals, rich in hearty carbohydrates, wholesome fats, and warming spices, we can invite a tapestry of flavours that sparks both appetite and spirit. These meals work not just to satiate but to invigorate, serving as a foundation of strength as we navigate the shorter days. Consider soup simmering with spices or an oven-roasted dish suffused with herbs—they're not just meals but rituals of warmth that fortify us against the cold. Through intentional eating, we're not just feeding our bodies; we're honouring the profound connection between nourishment and well-being that winter so poignantly highlights.

Warming Nutrients

The cold embrace of winter can often chill us to the bone, making it crucial to fuel our bodies with the warmth they crave. As the body battles against dropping temperatures, it seeks comfort not just from woollen layers but from the nutrients we consume. These warming nutrients are not just about filling our bellies; they are key players in sustaining energy, enhancing immunity, and fostering a sense of well-being throughout the frosty months.

Let's talk about whole grains, for instance. Whole grains such as oats, brown rice, and barley are rich in complex carbohydrates and serve as the foundational elements of a warming diet. When you consume them, these grains gradually release glucose into the bloodstream, providing a steady supply of energy that prevents those mid-afternoon slumps often exacerbated by winter's lethargy. Their fibre content also aids digestion, helping you feel fuller for longer and keeping your body's internal furnace burning steadily.

Spices and herbs can also be transformative during these cold months. Ginger, for instance, is renowned for its heat-inducing properties. A cup of ginger tea not only warms your hands but also invigorates your digestive system, reducing bloating and soothing nausea. It's these subtle enhancements that make spices and herbs indispensable allies in winter nutrition. Think of turmeric, with its anti-inflammatory prowess, or cinnamon, which can regulate blood sugar and add a hint of sweetness to your meals without relying on sugar.

On the topic of roots, vegetables like carrots, sweet potatoes, and beetroots are often overlooked despite their abundant benefits. These root vegetables are naturally dense in nutrients like beta-carotene and potassium. They can be roasted to perfection, bringing out their natural sweetness and deepening their warming effect. The slow release of their sugars during roasting not only caramelises them but also provides a sustained energy release, much like whole grains.

Protein, undisputedly, is another fundamental aspect of a warming diet. Whether derived from plant sources like lentils, chickpeas, and beans, or from lean meats and fish, protein aids in muscle repair and energy production. During winter when our physical activity levels might drop, maintaining muscle mass is crucial. A well-balanced intake of protein ensures that your body has what it needs to maintain its strength and vitality even as the temperature dips.

Fats are another crucial nutrient that shouldn't be sidelined. Healthy fats found in avocados, nuts, seeds, and oils like olive and coconut are vital for maintaining cell structure and producing energy. They act as a slow-burning fuel, perfect for enduring harsh weather. These fats are also fundamental for absorbing fat-soluble vitamins such as A, D, E, and K, which can play significant roles in immunity and bone health during the darker days of winter.

When embracing a nutrient-rich winter diet, it's important to recognize the role of **hydration**. Although it might not seem directly related to warmth, staying well-hydrated with fluids like herbal teas and broths is vital. These liquids help regulate body temperature and ensure that our physical systems function smoothly. Incorporating warming drinks like masala chai or matcha tea can provide a delightful, warming ritual while offering healthful benefits.

Moving beyond the functional aspects, food in winter takes on a deeper meaning. It becomes an exercise in mindfulness and gratitude. Preparing a warm, nourishing meal allows you to connect more profoundly with the ingredients. Winter invites you to slow down, savour each mouthful, and appreciate the warmth that radiates from a homemade stew or a bowl of spiced porridge. This mindful engagement isn't just about physical nourishment; it's also about fostering emotional warmth that radiates from within.

Lastly, don't overlook the social dimension of sharing meals. Gatherings around the dinner table, sharing stories and laughter over a comforting hotpot or a hearty soup, amplify the warmth we derive from our nutrition. It's not just the food that provides solace, but the connections we forge and the memories we create in these shared spaces.

Embrace the coming winter months with a heart full of warmth and a pantry stocked with these energy and wellness-enhancing nutrients. Each meal is an opportunity to nourish not just the body, but the soul. By weaving together these elements of warmth, vitality, and community, we lay a foundation for resilience, enabling us to thrive even as the snowflakes fall and the winds grow cold.

Creating Balanced Winter Meals

Winter is a season that nudges us to slow down, reflect, and rethink the ways we nourish ourselves. As the biting cold envelops us, our bodies naturally crave warmth and sustenance that go beyond mere comfort; they demand balance. Creating balanced winter meals isn't just about keeping hunger at bay, it's about cooking with intent and crafting dishes that fuel our vitality and inner warmth.

When the earth is blanketed in snow and the days are shorter, our food choices don't merely affect our physical energy, but also our emotional well-being. The primary goal of these meals is to provide a sense of equilibrium — a harmony that resonates within us, stoking the flames of resilience and serenity despite external chill. At its core, a balanced winter meal integrates a variety of food groups, each playing a distinctive role in fortifying our body against the season's challenges.

Whole grains are a cornerstone of any balanced meal, offering complex carbohydrates that release energy slowly, keeping us satiated and warm. Consider incorporating hearty grains such as quinoa, barley, or farro. These versatile grains can form the base of many dishes, adapting well to soups, stews, and salads. They're not only powerhouses of sustenance but also rich in essential minerals and vitamins like magnesium and B vitamins, which are crucial for energy metabolism.

Protein is another crucial component. During winter, boosting protein intake can aid in muscle maintenance and repair, especially if you're engaging in activities like winter sports or brisk walks. Lean meats such as chicken and turkey lend themselves beautifully to hearty winter dishes, with their ability to absorb and balance robust flavours. For plant-based diets, lentils, chickpeas, and beans are excellent alternatives, providing a protein punch with additional fibre benefits.

Then comes the aspect of incorporating stimulating spices and herbs. Culinary herbs such as rosemary, thyme, and sage hold aromatic qualities that enhance not just the taste, but also the nutritional value of winter meals. Indian-inspired spices like turmeric and ginger add warmth, aiding digestion and improving circulation, which is particularly beneficial during colder months. A pinch of cinnamon here and a sprinkle of nutmeg there can transform an ordinary dish into a comforting winter classic.

Vegetables, especially the root variety, are the unsung heroes of winter meals. Carrots, sweet potatoes, and parsnips, when roasted, take on a natural sweetness that feels like a warm embrace. These roots are rich in beta carotene and vitamin C, crucial for bolstering our immune system. Additionally, dark leafy greens like kale and Swiss chard should find a place at your table. Their vibrancy and high fibre content help in detoxifying and fortifying the body from within.

The inclusion of healthy fats is essential as well. Fatty acids found in foods like avocados, nuts, and olive oil support brain function and have anti-inflammatory properties. Incorporating these into meals can be as simple as drizzling some olive oil over a salad or munching on a handful of walnuts as a side treat.

Desserts in winter can be nourishing too, offering not just sweetness but an added layer of warmth. Consider poaching pears in red wine with cloves or baking apples with a hint of cinnamon. These treats bring comfort without the oversaturation of processed sugars, instead utilising the natural sweetness of fruits alongside the rich, warming elements of spices.

Balance also means mindfulness in meal preparation and consumption. The act of cooking itself can become a ritual of warmth — a momentary retreat from the whirlwind of daily life. Engaging with the process, from choosing seasonal ingredients to savouring the final meal, connects us more deeply to the nourishment we receive. It becomes an expression of gratitude for the sustenance that nature provides, even in its dormancy.

Beyond individual ingredients, balance in winter meals is also about portion control and ensuring a harmonious distribution of macronutrients. Eating in moderation without sacrificing satisfaction is key. Meals should leave you feeling invigorated rather than lethargic, energised rather than overly full.

Finally, let's not overlook the importance of staying hydrated. While it might not seem immediately relevant to meal balance, staying hydrated helps the body's metabolism and digestion, making sure the nutrients from all these carefully prepared meals are efficiently absorbed.

Combining these elements, you can create winter meals that are greater than the sum of their parts. Meals that warm not just your bones but also stir something deeper, a connection to the warmth within and to the nurturing gifts of nature. In crafting balanced winter meals, you foster an inner resilience and create a sanctuary of strength, one meal at a time.

Chapter 22:
Exploring Art and Creativity

Winter, with its hushed ambience and introspective allure, opens a portal to explore the depths of our creativity and the healing power of art. As the world outside hushes under a blanket of snow, it's the perfect time to delve into artistic pursuits that not only ignite our imagination but also soothe the soul. Engaging in creative workshops, whether painting the shimmering contrast of winter landscapes or crafting heartfelt illustrations, can serve as a balm for the spirit. This chapter encourages you to immerse yourself in art as winter therapy, an antidote to the season's grey days, and a means to cultivate a radiant inner warmth. Whether you're painting, crafting, or attending pottery classes, these creative endeavours inspire joy, foster mindfulness, and nurture our resilient core. Art beckons with an invitation to express, explore, and enrich our lives, enhancing our capacity for well-being during the winter months.

Art as a Winter Therapy

Amidst the short days and long nights of winter, art emerges as a warm beacon, providing solace and a therapeutic refuge from the chill. Engaging in creative activities doesn't just pass the time; it nurtures spiritual and emotional well-being in unique ways. When snowflakes dance in the air and icy winds creep through cracks, transformative power lies within every brushstroke, sketch, and splash of colour. Art, in its many forms, offers a sanctuary for the heart and mind during the winter months.

Winter days can feel isolating, with our spirits wrapped tightly in layers of cold indifference. Art breaks through these barriers, connecting us to ourselves and the world around us. It enables us to express emotions we can't quite put into words and discovers parts of ourselves that lie dormant in the warm months. When working with paint, clay, or textiles, we embark on a journey of self-expression that can be both revealing and liberating.

For many, the strokes of a paintbrush or the rhythm of poetry offer a meditative experience. Winter invites us to slow down, and in doing so, the practice of creating art becomes a deliberate act of mindfulness. Paying attention to the minutiae — the way light hits an object, the subtle blending of colours, or the texture of a charcoal line — when we're this conscious, it quiets the mind and centres the soul.

Art as Therapy

The therapeutic value of art reaches across ages and personal experiences. For some, it's a playful release of energy; for others, a deep and reflective practice. Those wrestling with the weight of winter often find a reprieve in creative expression. Crafting, drawing, or painting allows emotions to flow unhindered, offering a canvas for processing feelings that can become overwhelming in the winter's hush.

Furthermore, art provides a mode of communication where words fail. It bridges gaps in emotional expression, allowing us to externalise what's inside. Art therapy has proven its worth in reducing anxiety, alleviating stress, and even assisting with depression. The hands-on nature of creating something tangible can offer comfort and promote a sense of achievement, lifting spirits one brushstroke at a time.

Creating Together

While solitary art-making carries its own reward, collaborating with others can be equally enriching. Winter workshops and classes can bring people together, fostering a sense of community and shared purpose. Groups focusing on art as therapy allow participants to bond over their creations and offer support and encouragement to one another. These gatherings become a warm respite from the cold, galvanising human connection and creativity.

Art encourages us to see the world through each other's eyes, breaking down barriers that might otherwise stand stark in an otherwise isolated season. Sharing the creative process builds trust and solidarity, fostering relationships that provide warmth in the frostiest days. Whether in local community centres or online spaces, creative workshops become havens where inspiration blooms.

Embracing Different Mediums

The beauty of art as a therapy lies in its versatility. Not restricted to traditional mediums, it encourages exploration and experimentation. Some find solace in the tactile qualities of clay, shaping forms that mirror the fluidity of their thoughts. Others may prefer the immediacy of photography, capturing moments of beauty in the starkness of a winter landscape.

Textiles, too, offer a rich tapestry for creativity, with knitting or weaving providing rhythmic satisfaction. The repetitive motions can be soothing, serving as a form of meditation while producing something beautiful and useful. These forms of art harness the power of touch, texture, and movement, rooting us in the physical world while allowing the mind to drift into realms of imagination.

Digital media expands the reach of art therapy, providing access to creative tools that can be used anywhere, anytime. Platforms for digital creativity empower users to edit photos, produce music, or design graphics, all from the comfort of their home. These tools democratise creativity, enabling anyone with a smartphone or computer to explore art as a tool for well-being.

The Inspirational Element

Art's potential to inspire is heightened during winter. The snow-laden landscape transforms the world into a canvas of contrast, where bare branches etch patterns against a blanket of white. Inspiration is found in the way frost clings to the windowpane or the muted glow of a winter sunset. Artists often find their surroundings mirrored back through their work, reinterpreting the season's chill into vibrant expressions of colour and form.

For those who embrace journals and sketchbooks, drawing inspiration from the intimate moments of winter provides an ongoing project. A daily sketch or entry captures the ephemeral aspects of the season — a practice of observing and documenting the subtle changes that might otherwise go unnoticed.

The quietude of winter offers a palette of subtle hues and transitional light that presents both challenge and opportunity for artists. The stark beauty of the season invites contemplation and reflection, offering a unique muse for those willing to see it. When immersed in creative projects, the short, grey days seem to stretch into timeless moments, freeing us from winter's constraints.

Nurturing through Creativity

Engaging in art as therapy during winter establishes routines that nurture and sustain. Setting aside dedicated time for creative pursuits not only provides structure but acts as an anchor, grounding us against seasonal turbulence. Whether creating art alone in a quiet corner or surrounded by like-minded people, this practice offers moments of stillness and focus amidst the season's cacophony.

Turning to art in difficult times reminds us of the resilience and beauty that reside within us. It offers not just a distraction, but a meaningful encounter with our inner selves. As winter unfolds, creativity becomes a steadfast companion — a testament to human ingenuity, adaptability, and the relentless pursuit of warmth amidst the cold.

Embracing art as a winter therapy is more than just a casual pastime; it's a powerful means of fortifying one's emotional and spiritual resilience. It's about turning the season's introspective pause into a flourishing of self-expression, reconnecting with the world and oneself. In this light, art transforms wintertime into a canvas on which we paint our own stories of resilience and hope.

Engaging in Creative Workshops

As the chill of winter encourages us to draw inward, it also presents the perfect opportunity to explore our creative sides. Engaging in creative workshops isn't just a way to pass the time; it's an invitation to ignite something dormant within us. In the heart of winter, when the world outside may seem monochrome and still, these workshops offer bursts of colour and movement, transforming our inner landscapes. They serve as beacons of light in the longer evenings, drawing people together to share, learn, and create.

The beauty of creative workshops lies in their diversity. From pottery to painting, writing to weaving, there's something for everyone. Whether you're an expert or a novice, the workshop setting is designed to nurture your creative spirit in an environment free from judgment. The emphasis is on exploration and expression rather than perfection. This release from the pressure of perfect results can be incredibly liberating. Participating in such activities often uncovers unexpected talents and surprising insights about oneself.

Consider a pottery workshop, where your hands are your primary tools and clay is your medium. Here, the tactile experience of shaping earth into form is profoundly grounding. The rhythmic motion of the potter's wheel, combined with the malleability of the clay, connects us to ancient traditions while also serving as a form of moving meditation. Each piece that emerges is unique, carrying the imprint of its creator's mood, touch, and energy. This form of artistry harnesses the heart of slow creation, allowing participants to savour each step of the process.

Residing in the written word, writing workshops provide an alternate canvas. Through prompts, guided exercises, and the sharing of prose or poetry, individuals can find their narrative voice. Such environments foster deep reflection and community support, making it easier to experience cathartic release. Winter's quietude offers time for journaling, capturing the cadence of one's inner thoughts, which may otherwise remain unwritten. Writing workshops cultivate a space where personal stories are honoured, weaving individual tales into a collective tapestry.

Ultimately, the magic of creative workshops is in their ability to harness imagination, transporting us beyond the constraints of daily life. The very act of creating fosters a sense of presence, a connection to the now. Engaging in these activities allows individuals to explore different facets of their personalities, nurture their well-being, and enhance their mental resilience. By dedicating time and space to these creative pursuits, we give ourselves permission to dream and discover.

Music and sound workshops perfect this connection while appealing to our auditory senses. Whether learning an instrument or participating in a chant circle, sound provides a unique way to express creativity. Musical abilities aren't required; even simply exploring various sounds or beats can invigorate the soul. These experiences foster focus and flow state, where time seems to melt away, leaving us with a feeling of deep satisfaction and connection. Music and sound have a profound ability to bring people together, uniting different voices in harmonious expression.

Workshops also offer the prospect of communal creativity—an intimate, human experience that is especially treasured in the colder months, when social isolation can intensify. The act of creating alongside others, sharing insights and experiences, weaves a network of support and solidarity. In such spaces, creative energies are reflected and amplified, sparking new ideas and forging deeper bonds. This sense of belonging can be a powerful antidote to winter's solitude, providing warmth of heart and spirit.

One may find wonder in craft workshops, where hands take on the task of bringing ideas into the tangible realm. Textile arts like knitting or crocheting produce cosy items that bring immediate warmth. The rhythmic actions soothe the mind, much like rocking a cradle, creating a tranquil state where stress dissipates, and creativity flows. These crafts, with roots tied to tradition, imbue a sense of continuity and connection with the past, harmoniously blending mindfulness with skill.

Celebrating creativity can extend beyond the individual, impacting the community at large. Hosting or attending open workshops helps spread the joy of creation. Local artists, craftspeople, and creatives often run sessions that open doors to new skills and connections. Supporting these local enthusiasts not only enriches personal creativity but fosters cultural resilience, encouraging economic reciprocity and fostering a sense of community spirit. Such networks can be vital in maintaining local culture, offering a sensory richness that lingers long after the sessions have ended.

In a world where time proficiently marches forward, creative workshops urge us to slow down, to savour and appreciate the beauty of the process. Engagement in these activities throughout the winter months crafts a tapestry of warmth, resilience, and wellbeing. As our creations take shape, we remind ourselves of our innate ability to adapt and evolve, mirroring the subtle transformations of winter leading to spring's renewal. Let these workshops be a cornerstone of making this season not just one of endurance, but of blooming creativity.

As you open yourself to these experiences, keep in mind that the spectrum of creativity is vast—no matter where your interests lie, there's a workshop waiting to infuse your winter with vibrancy and warmth. Embark on this creative journey, not for the pursuit of greatness but for the sheer joy of creation. These labs of imagination and skill will accompany you through the cold season, knitting warmth and wonder into the very fabric of your winter.

Chapter 23:
Reconnecting with Nature

In the heart of winter, where the world appears hushed and blanketed in stillness, a profound opportunity arises to reconnect with nature. This season encourages us to venture outdoors, embracing the crisp air that invigorates the spirit and sharpens the senses. Whether walking along frost-laden paths or marvelling at the subtle dance of bare branches, there's a quiet magic that beckons reflection and appreciation. Reconnecting with nature doesn't stop at the door; by welcoming natural elements into our homes, like evergreen sprigs or pinecones, we create sanctuaries of calm and resilience. These connections remind us of nature's enduring cycles and our place within them, nurturing a sense of balance and well-being. In nature's gentle embrace, we find timeless wisdom and the invitation to slow down, observe, and simply be.

Nature Walks and Observations

As winter embraces the land with its frosty touch, the natural world offers a quiet invitation to step outside and reconnect. The cool, crisp air fills your lungs, awakening your senses in a way that only the chill of winter can. Nature walks during this time offer a unique tapestry of experiences that may not be seen in any other season. Each step through snow-blanketed trails or frost-kissed paths allows us to observe the subtle shifts and transformations that nature undergoes.

The winter landscape is a study in contrasts. Bare branches etch intricate patterns against the grey skies, revealing the skeletal beauty of trees hidden during leafier months. Each footprint left behind in the fresh snow speaks of who or what has ventured that way, adding an element of mystery and discovery. These imprints invite questions: was it a fox on its nightly hunt or a deer traversing quiet forests? Observing these details not only anchors us to the present moment but also nourishes a deep connection to the earth and its rhythms.

In the quietude, nature's subtler aspects become more pronounced. The rustle of a small bird in the underbrush or the gentle drip of melting icicles can seem amplified in the stillness. There's a meditative quality to winter walks, where each crunch through the snow can match the steady inhale and exhale of your breath. Taking time to pause, we notice the opportunity to reflect not only on our surroundings but also on our own inner landscapes. With the world stripped of its usual grandeur, there's a clarity and sincerity to winter observations that mirrors our quest for inner warmth and resilience during these months.

Winter's palette is understated yet profound. The muted tones of browns, greys, and whites create a subtle beauty all their own. Each grey sky and snowy field offer a blank canvas that invites imagination and introspection. You might catch sight of a cardinal's brilliant red against a snowy backdrop or the soft green of an evergreen crowned with snow, these splashes of colour feel almost poetic. Such encounters remind us of the resilience and persistence of life, even in the harshest conditions, and encourage us to find beauty in the simplicity of the present moment.

In some regions, winter brings with it migratory birds, a fitting metaphor for life's cyclic nature. Witnessing these visitors offers a sense of continuity and temporal connection to other natural cycles. This season also offers the opportunity to become familiar with local species that remain, observing how they've adapted to their environment. Whether it's the sight of a hawk perched royally against a snow-laden branch or the persistent chirp of a chickadee, these moments highlight the interconnectedness of all living things.

Even the ground beneath our feet tells its own winter story. With the thick carpet of leaves gone, the contours of the land become more apparent. Hills and valleys seem steeper, streams and rivers become clearer, their icy surfaces mirrored reflections of the surrounding landscapes. The crunch of snow or the slip of ice underfoot brings an awareness to each step that is both grounding and exhilarating.

For those who seek to deepen their engagement with the natural world during winter, note-taking can become an extension of your observations. Carry a small notebook to jot down what you see, hear, and feel. Such practices sharpen your awareness and bring mindfulness into your walks. Sketching a quick outline of a leafless tree or writing a poem inspired by the gentle snowfall further cultivates a rich appreciation for the season and its unique offerings.

Consider pairing your walks with gentle practices such as mindfulness or yoga. Pausing to breathe deeply and stretch amidst the enveloping beauty of nature can enhance both physical and mental well-being. Letting go of distractions, your senses awaken to the rhythm of nature, which, in turn, fosters a deeper connection within yourself. This integration of movement and environment sets the stage for renewed vitality and resilience, essential components of navigating the winter months with grace.

Yet, nature's generosity in winter doesn't stop at beauty alone. Winter walks can also serve as informal teachers of resilience, patience, and change. As we watch a tree unwavering against strong winds or a frozen pond patiently awaiting the thaw, we're reminded of our own capacity for endurance and growth. Such moments invite reflection on how we, like the natural world, can adapt to and flourish amid life's inevitable challenges.

Beyond individual reflection, nature walks can also be a shared experience, offering opportunities to connect with loved ones. Walking in silence alongside a friend or family member, or sharing thoughts inspired by nature's artistry, can foster deeper bonds. These shared moments offer warmth that extends beyond physical realms, nurturing connections that thrive even in the coldest months.

Ultimately, embracing winter through nature walks and observations rewards us with a richer understanding of our environment and, in turn, ourselves. As you employ all your senses to explore the world around you, a quiet transformation takes place. You gain an informed appreciation of what it means to be part of this vast, interconnected web of life. So, as the season unfolds, venture out onto those frost-covered paths. Let the serene winter landscape guide you, offering peace and insights as you reconnect with nature and your own inner being.

Bringing Nature Indoors

Bringing the natural world into our homes during the winter months can create a sanctuary that nurtures our well-being and rejuvenates the spirit. As the days grow shorter and temperatures drop, an internal landscape can thrive just as vibrantly as the one beyond our doors. It invites us to explore the rich textures, calming colours, and sensory experiences of nature without stepping outside. There's something inherently soothing about surrounding ourselves with greenery and natural elements that breathe life into our spaces, encouraging an atmosphere of warmth even amidst the frostiest of days.

Indoor plants are a wonderful way to infuse a sense of the outdoors into our homes. They act as natural air purifiers, improving indoor air quality while delighting the senses with their beauty. Choose plants that thrive in indoor winter conditions such as peace lilies, snake plants, and English ivy. Their ease of care makes them perfect companions during the season. Arranging these plants in areas where natural light filters in — perhaps near a windowsill or in a sun-drenched nook — can maximise their growth and remind us of nature's resilience.

Incorporating natural materials into home decor is another effective way to feel connected to nature. Wood, stone, and natural fibres can be woven into our spaces through furniture, flooring, or decorative elements. Imagine a soft wool throw draped over a wooden chair, or pebbles gathered in a bowl on a tabletop. These tactile elements invite a closeness to the earth and imbue our interior environments with a grounding energy. They evoke peacefulness and remind us of the simplicity found in nature's designs.

While the visible beauty of nature is uplifting, don't underestimate the power of natural aromas to transform a space. Essential oils and natural candles in scents like pine, cedar, and eucalyptus can evoke the great outdoors, creating a sensory experience that calms the mind and refreshes the spirit. Aromatherapy not only adds warmth to your home but can also be a form of self-care during the winter months, helping to balance mood and restore energy.

Experimenting with seasonal décor, reflecting the outdoors, also serves to bring nature inside. Consider creating displays using branches, pinecones, or dried flowers gathered on a crisp winter walk. These organic decorations can evolve throughout the season, as nature itself continually changes. Such displays not only connect us to the rhythms of the natural world but also offer a creative outlet during the quieter months, encouraging mindfulness as we mindfully arrange each element.

Moreover, the presence of nature within our homes can serve as gentle reminders of the cycles all beings go through. Just as plants flourish, wither, and bloom again, we too undergo phases of rest and renewal. This consciousness can be comforting, instilling patience and acceptance towards ourselves during times when we feel dormant, knowing that this too is a part of life's natural ebb and flow.

It's important to create moments to engage with the natural elements in our living spaces. Mindfully water your plants, prune their leaves, and observe their quiet growth around you. This act of care and attention fosters a relationship with the living elements of your home and kindles a deeper appreciation for the delicate balance and beauty found in nature. Indeed, this practice can amplify our capacity for gratitude, inviting us to marvel at the small miracles unfolding in the coziness of our homes.

Beyond aesthetics and atmosphere, fostering an indoor relationship with nature can have profound impacts on our mental and emotional well-being. Studies suggest that simply being in the presence of plants can reduce stress, lower blood pressure, and improve overall mental health. As the winter months can sometimes challenge our mental resilience, these natural remedies become even more vital.

Finally, cultivating nature indoors is about crafting an experience that aligns with our personal aesthetics and needs. It's about finding joy and serenity in the layers of life we invite within our walls. While our world outdoors slows in winter, our indoor sanctuary remains a vibrant testament to the continuity and ever-present beauty of nature. Let it be a source of inspiration and comfort, reminding us of the interconnection between all living things and enriching our journey inward during this reflective season.

Chapter 24:
Setting Winter Goals

As the frost blankets the earth, inviting a season of stillness and introspection, setting winter goals becomes an exercise in aligning our intentions with nature's quiet pause. This time of year offers a unique opportunity to recalibrate our aspirations, mindful of the rhythms that encourage both rest and renewal. Within this reflective framework, we can craft goals that nurture our inner warmth and resilience, gently challenging ourselves while honouring our need for tranquillity. By choosing aspirations that harmonise with the winter's embrace, such as deepening mindfulness practices or exploring creative outlets, we set the stage for a transformative journey into the new year. Keep the progress steady and intentions flexible, allowing for the ebb and flow that accompany the season's changes. Embracing this intuitive approach not only enhances our growth but also fortifies the spirit, lighting a path that merges ambition with the soulful peace of winter's grace.

Goal-Setting Strategies

Winter, with its serene landscapes and quietude, offers a unique canvas for introspection and the setting of meaningful goals. Unlike the bustling warmth of summer, winter invites us to turn inwards, to reflect, and to consciously set intentions that align with our innermost desires. Goal-setting during this season isn't just about ticking boxes or fulfilling obligations; it's about fostering personal growth and embracing change, drawing warmth from our achievements as days grow colder.

One effective strategy for setting winter goals is aligning them with the natural rhythm of the season. Winter is a time of rest, a pause in the cycle of nature. By acknowledging this, you can set goals that focus on rest, rejuvenation, and preparation for the vibrant activity of spring. Consider what aspects of your life need replenishment or a gentle nurturing touch. Perhaps it's time to focus on self-care, developing a meditation practice, or reigniting a passion that was set aside during busier months.

Another technique involves breaking down larger goals into manageable, bite-sized steps. This method is particularly beneficial during winter when energy levels may fluctuate. Small, consistent actions can build momentum, boosting your confidence and creating a sense of achievement. Starting each day with a simple intention can keep you aligned and focused, lighting the path towards larger aspirations.

Creating anticipation and excitement around your goals is essential too. While winter is a time for introspection, it shouldn't be devoid of joy or enthusiasm. Visualise your goals vividly. What will achieving them feel like? Sketch mental pictures of success and happiness. Use tools like vision boards or journals to keep these images tangible. Such creativity can bridge the gap between imagination and reality, propelling you towards your intentions with zeal and purpose.

Moreover, personal reflection is a cornerstone of effective winter goal-setting strategies. Taking time to journal or meditate can offer insights into what's truly important to you. Reflect on past winters. What lessons have you learned? What goals did you achieve—or not—and why? Such reflections are invaluable as they provide a firm foundation from which you can reach new heights.

Accountability is another powerful tool in the goal-setting arsenal. Sharing your goals with someone you trust can provide motivation and a sense of responsibility. Whether it's a close friend, a family member, or a community group, having someone to discuss your progress with can make the journey less daunting and more rewarding. These connections can offer perspectives you hadn't considered, enriching your path to success.

Winter is also a fitting time to practice gratitude, an often overlooked component of goal-setting. By recognising and appreciating the small victories along the way, you reinforce motivation and encourage a positive mindset. This appreciation fosters resilience and helps you stay grounded, particularly when faced with challenges. Keep a gratitude journal where you jot down achievements and highlight personal progress, no matter how minute.

Flexibility in your approach to goal-setting is equally important. While structure is beneficial, rigidity can lead to frustration, especially in winter when plans might need to change due to unforeseen circumstances. Be willing to adapt your goals and methods if they no longer serve you. Flexibility allows for a more organic progression towards your aspirations, accommodating the ebb and flow of life during these colder months.

Lastly, consider the timing of your goals. While some goals may naturally align with the holiday season, others might be more suited to the quieter, introspective moments of January and February. Use this seasonal framework to prioritise and schedule your endeavours. Aligning your goals with the calendar can provide a sense of direction, ensuring that you remain focused throughout the winter months.

Embracing these strategies can transform your winter goal-setting from a mundane task into an enriching practice of self-discovery and empowerment. Through thoughtful goal-setting, you not only nurture your inner strength but also lay a foundation for a year filled with warmth, balance, and resilience. As the snow blankets the earth, may your dreams and desires take root, strong and ready to blossom with the arrival of spring. The work you do now in setting your goals can lead you toward a season of growth and renewal, underscoring the profound interplay between introspection and action that winter so beautifully supports.

Tracking Progress

Setting winter goals is only the beginning of your journey towards cultivating a season of warmth and well-being. To ensure these goals aren't just aspirations but realities, tracking your progress becomes crucial. Each step you take towards fulfilling your winter goals can strengthen your inner resilience and harmony, offering a sense of accomplishment and clarity amidst the cold months.

One of the most effective approaches to tracking progress is through regular reflection. Weekly or even daily check-ins can provide insight into how far you've come and what areas might need more attention. A simple notebook or digital journal can be your ally in this process. By noting down achievements and challenges, you create a tangible record of your journey, making it easier to see patterns and shifts in your path.

Set aside time each week to examine your progress—this can be during a quiet Sunday morning or a reflective Friday evening. Consider not just the goals you've ticked off but also the feelings these achievements elicit. Reflect on questions like, "What have I learned this week?" or "How has working towards my goals improved my sense of well-being?" Such questions delve deeper than surface-level progress, encouraging a more profound connection with your journey.

Incorporating visual aids like progress charts or vision boards can be particularly motivational. Colourful charts can serve as a visual testament to your efforts, while vision boards can keep your overarching objectives in view. Whether you sketch, doodle, or paste, these tools can breathe life into your ambitions, adding a creative flair to the otherwise analytical process of tracking progress.

Sharing your journey with a trusted friend or a supportive group can also be immensely powerful. Engaging others in your progress can provide external feedback, encouragement, and perhaps even a fresh perspective on your goals. Another's insight could be just what you need to adjust your course or celebrate successes you didn't acknowledge for yourself.

Beyond the tangible measures and shared reflections, internal mindfulness acts as a compass, guiding you towards genuine progress. Practicing mindfulness—whether through meditation, breathing exercises, or simply moments of stillness—centres your focus on the present. This awareness allows you to assess your progress more holistically, balancing the mind's chatter against your heart's quiet truth.

Recognise that progress isn't always linear. Winter's unpredictable rhythm—its oscillation between serene snowfalls and unpredictable storms—mirrors the nature of our progress. Some weeks might feel slow, while others are filled with leaps forward. Embrace these fluctuations with kindness and curiosity, understanding that each step, no matter how small, fuels your overall growth.

Adjusting goals as you progress is also a critical aspect of tracking. As you evolve, so too might your desires and circumstances. An adaptable approach allows your winter goals to remain relevant and realistic. Regularly revisit and refine your objectives; this ensures they continue to support your overarching vision of inner warmth and well-being.

Acknowledge and celebrate milestones, no matter their size. Each achievement is a testament to your dedication and perseverance.

Celebrations can be as simple as enjoying a quiet cup of tea while watching the snow fall or engaging in a heartfelt conversation with a loved one. These moments of joy and recognition can bolster your motivation, propelling you forward with renewed energy.

Lastly, view the process of tracking as an art rather than a rigid system. Allow creativity and intuition to guide how you monitor your journey. This organic approach can make the experience more engaging and fulfilling, transforming goal-setting into an integral part of your winter's narrative.

As we explore the essence of tracking progress, we remember that this practice is less about reaching a final destination and more about deeply engaging with the journey itself. In doing so, we cultivate a profound sense of self-awareness and resilience, preparing our hearts for the eventual return of spring. Progress, like winter, is a season—a transformative cycle that fosters growth in its unique, introspective way.

Chapter 25:
Embracing Change and
Transformation

As the stark beauty of winter envelops us, it's a time to embrace the profound potential for change and transformation nestled within the season's quietude. Winter, with its bare landscapes and shorter days, offers a reflective space that encourages us to look inward and consider the personal growth journeys we can embark upon. It's a powerful period to shed old patterns and make room for new habits that better serve our well-being. Transformation is not merely about drastic shifts but about small, intentional steps that lead to lasting change. By honouring this process, we prepare ourselves for the inevitable rebirth of spring, both ready and resilient for the new opportunities it brings. The rhythm of winter teaches patience and the value of gradual progress, reminding us that every end is also a fresh beginning. While nature is in its dormancy, our inner worlds can bloom with insights, setting the foundation for the vibrant renewal of our lives.

Personal Growth in Winter

Winter, with its enveloping chill and serene landscapes, offers a unique invitation for personal growth. It's a season that naturally encourages introspection, providing a backdrop for profound transformation if we're open to it. While on the surface, winter may seem a time of dormancy, beneath the frosty exterior lies an opportunity for renewal and self-discovery. This season, often misunderstood as bleak, can serve as a powerful catalyst for inner evolution, encouraging us to peel away layers and engage deeply with ourselves.

Amidst the short days and long nights, winter gently persuades us to slow down. This deceleration is not just physical but mental too, offering space to examine our life's narrative deeply. It's a time for reflection, where one can explore past achievements and setbacks, not with judgment, but with the intent to understand and learn. In the quietude of winter, there's a chance to listen to our inner voice—a voice that often gets drowned out in the hustle and bustle of warmer months.

The stillness of winter provides an ideal setting for setting intentions and contemplating life's bigger questions. It's not about grand resolutions but about small, intentional shifts. With clarity derived from self-reflection, we can discern what truly matters and align our actions accordingly. This process requires honesty and patience, but slowly, it nurtures a sense of purpose and direction, strengthening our resolve to cultivate the changes we wish to see in ourselves.

Winter's embrace can also be a period to develop resilience and adaptability. These darker, colder months teach us about endurance and the importance of internal fortitude. When external conditions are harsh, we often turn inwards, fostering an inner strength that transcends seasonal boundaries. This resilience, once cultivated in winter, sustains us throughout the year, empowering us to navigate both life's expected transitions and unforeseen challenges.

Personal growth during winter isn't just about introspection, though. It's also about embracing new habits that affirm and enhance our well-being. The crisp, cold air beckons us outside, urging us to engage with the natural world. Whether it's winter walks that clear the mind or serene outdoor solitude that brings peace, nature provides a therapeutic escape from the confines of everyday concerns. These activities allow the rejuvenation of the body and mind, creating a foundation for holistic well-being.

Engaged creativity can be another avenue for growth in winter. When the sun sets early, and evenings stretch out before us, there's a beautiful opportunity to explore creative pursuits that bring joy and fulfilment. Whether it's painting, writing, or engaging in expressive arts, the act of creation can serve as a meditation, a way to process emotions, and a path towards self-discovery. Each brushstroke or written word becomes a dialogue with the self, revealing insights and sparking new ideas.

As we nurture creativity, winter also encourages us to embrace learning and education. With more time spent indoors, there's an opportunity to dive into new topics or revisit neglected interests. Whether it's learning a new language, delving into historical literature, or participating in online courses, expanding our knowledge opens horizons and enriches our understanding of the world and ourselves. This intellectual nourishment harmonises with winter's theme of growth and transformation, easing our journey towards self-improvement.

Moreover, personal growth in winter can involve strengthening our relationships. The tight-knit gatherings typical of winter months remind us of the warmth that connection brings. Engaging deeply with family and friends, whether through shared meals or intimate conversations, enhances our empathy and understanding. These connections act as mirrors, reflecting our growth and encouraging us to continue evolving, not in isolation but within a web of interconnectedness.

Ultimately, personal growth in winter requires a degree of courage—to face the cold, both literal and metaphorical, and to venture into the depths of the self. Yet, it's within this chill that a robust inner fire can be ignited. By embracing the lessons of the season, we foster a resilience and warmth that not only sustains us during winter but empowers us as spring arrives, bringing with it its own opportunities for rebirth and new beginnings. The transformation experienced during these cold months is, therefore, both a conclusion and a prelude, as we prepare to carry forward what we have learned into the coming seasons.

Spring Preparation

As winter begins its gradual retreat, the world around us stirs from its months-long slumber. There's an undeniable magic in the air as daylight extends its reach, and you can almost hear the gentle whisper of spring urging its way through the frost. Embracing this transition isn't just about accepting nature's metamorphosis but also about readying our minds and bodies for the warmth and renewal spring promises.

Preparation for spring is not merely a physical act; it's a mindset. Picture the gentle awakening of the trees, the tentative emergence of the first crocus, and how these herald a time of growth and opportunity. Similarly, our own inner transformation should be fostered by a conscious readiness to welcome what lies ahead. Just as we have learned to adapt and find comfort in winter, we must also open ourselves to the flourishing energy of spring.

Now, what does it mean to prepare for spring? Much like tidying a garden after months of winter wear, preparing for the change involves a bit of cleaning and renewal. Consider using this time to declutter your living spaces, allowing light to enter more freely, and reimagining your environment to reflect the vivacity of the season. Decluttering isn't just about removing physical items; it's about creating a mental space free of clutter, a space that invites creativity and clarity.

Think about how you can bring elements of the burgeoning season into your home. Swap out heavy blankets for lighter throws, introduce fresh colours reminiscent of blossoms and new growth, and perhaps try your hand at planting herbs or flowers to celebrate the new season. These seemingly small acts can have a substantial impact on your overall well-being, as they symbolise the new beginnings inherent to spring.

As spring beckons, there also lies the opportunity to reflect on personal growth. Winter, with its introspective qualities, has laid a foundation upon which new aspirations can be built. Take a moment to revisit any goals or intentions set earlier and assess their development. Spring offers a platform for progression, a time to sow seeds of ambition and nurture them as daylight increases and nature rejuvenates.

Furthermore, consider how diet and self-care rituals might shift in harmony with the seasonal change. Lighter, refreshing foods can begin to replace the hearty meals of winter, reflecting the fresh produce and vibrant flavours that become available. Embrace an adaptive routine that allows for more outdoor activities as the weather becomes milder, welcoming the invigorating energy that comes with it.

Spring preparation isn't confined to individuals; it's a collective transformation. Engage with your community and think about how to foster connections that encourage mutual growth and support. It might be the ideal time to collaborate on community projects, initiate a garden club, or find new ways to spend time outdoors with friends and family.

As spring approaches, recognise the empowerment that comes from embracing change. Change isn't something to be feared; it's an essential part of growth. Just as the ice melts and rivers begin to flow with renewed vigour, we too can follow nature's example and embrace transformation with openness and enthusiasm.

Let spring's arrival inspire your personal journey of evolution and warmth. As nature unfolds its intricate tapestry of greens and blooms, allow yourself the same capacity for renewal and growth. Remember, the preparation you undertake now sets the tone for a vibrant and fulfilling season ahead.

Conclusion

As the final chapter of our journey through the winter season draws to a close, it is essential to recognise the power of embracing this time for self-development and reflection. Despite winter's reputation for bleakness, it holds unique opportunities for personal growth, well-being, and introspection. We've journeyed together, exploring ways to cultivate warmth and resilience amidst the cold, and now, as you stand at the threshold of spring, it's time to reflect on the lessons learned and the transformations undergone.

Throughout the pages of this book, we've uncovered the magic that lies in winter's quietude. The serenity that this season can bring is unmatched, allowing us moments of stillness often lost in the frenetic pace of modern life. By adopting a slower, more mindful approach, we've discovered how winter's rest can fortify the spirit and rejuvenate the mind. This period of gentle dormancy encourages us to pause, to breathe, and ultimately, to grow.

Through nourishing foods and warming rituals, winter becomes not a barrier to overcome but a friend to embrace. We've explored seasonal ingredients, rich with nutrients, that fuel our bodies and spirit whilst keeping the colder elements at bay. These culinary delights are more than meals; they are invitations to savour each bite, experience vitality, and nourish from within. Likewise, the warmth of a cosy home and the comforting smell of aromatherapy oils create a sanctuary for rest and reflection.

Our bodies have been revered as temples needing care amid the harshness of winter. Skin, often vulnerable in these months, has been given loving attention and protection against elements that strip away moisture and vitality. Ritualistic bathing practices have reminded us of the importance of self-care, turning ordinary routines into moments of profound connection with oneself. Meanwhile, fostering mental resilience through meditation and positive mindset practices has equipped us to weather life's storms with equanimity and grace.

The social connections we nurture in winter are vital threads in the tapestry of well-being. Winter is the perfect time to gather and celebrate with loved ones, fostering those bonds that sustain us. Through creative gatherings and genuine interactions, we ensure that our hearts remain warmed not only by fireplaces but by friendships and shared laughter.

In addition, exploring the benefits of light and sound has brought a transformative element to our winter experience. The role of light, natural or enhanced, has illuminated dark days, providing a necessary counterbalance to the season's dimness. The sounds of winter, whether in playlists that lift the mood or the power of silence, have added a rich texture to these months, helping to soothe the soul.

As we balance our work and leisure, we learn that winter doesn't have to hinder our creativity but can instead be a muse that nurtures and inspires new hobbies and forms of expression. Winter travel may bring adventure and new perspectives, while creative expression keeps our spirits alight as the days grow shorter. Spiritual practices remind us of the fire within that is never extinguished, even by winter's longest nights.

Most importantly, this journey has taught us to embrace change and see winter as more than just a transition. It's a time of personal growth, a preparation for spring, where we apply the lessons of acceptance, gratitude, and mindfulness to the broader canvas of life. As you step forward, carrying these insights in your heart, may you find that the gifts of winter echo throughout all seasons, nurturing a life of balance, warmth, and well-being year-round.

Appendix A:
Appendix

This appendix serves as a comprehensive resource for anyone seeking solace and personal growth throughout the winter months. We've gathered a selection of valuable resources designed to help you nurture well-being and resilience as you embrace winter. From nourishing recipes that warm the soul to curated reading lists that inspire introspection, the tools provided here aim to enhance your journey towards harmony. Whether you're delving into new self-care techniques or exploring time-honoured traditions, this section is crafted to offer support and inspiration. Let these resources guide you towards creating a season imbued with warmth, balance, and vitality, encouraging you to step into each new day with renewed energy and positivity.

Resources for Winter Wellness

As winter envelops us in its frosty embrace, finding resources that foster warmth and well-being becomes essential. This section offers a collection of valuable tools and materials carefully chosen to enhance your winter wellness journey. Whether you're seeking physical comfort, mental clarity, or spiritual nourishment, these resources serve as a companion in navigating the season with grace and vitality.

One of the most accessible resources is the power of music—an uplifting melody can transform a grey winter afternoon into a radiant moment of joy. Consider creating a winter playlist that resonates with your spirit. Include a blend of soulful tunes, energising beats, or tranquil melodies that suit different times of the day. Music has the ability to enhance mood, inspire creativity, and offer solace when days seem long and nights are cold.

Books, too, provide a refuge of warmth and wisdom. This season, delve into works that explore themes of resilience, mindfulness, and personal growth. Titles focusing on embracing the seasons, cultivating inner calm, or even fictional tales set in enchanting winter landscapes can serve as both a comforting escape and an insightful guide.

Those yearning for a more tactile experience might find comfort in creative pursuits. Crafting provides a physical outlet for expression and mindfulness. Engage in projects that utilise natural materials, like pine cones, dried flowers, or wool. Not only do they bring a piece of the outdoors in, but these activities can also foster a meditative state, allowing for a deeper connection with the present moment.

In terms of physical health, herbal remedies play a crucial role in winter wellness. Books on herbal medicine can be invaluable as references for creating soothing teas and infusions that boost immunity and alleviate winter ailments. Herbs such as echinacea, ginger, and elderberry are acclaimed for their immune-enhancing properties, providing natural support throughout the colder months.

Technological aids like apps designed for guided meditation and mindfulness can be beneficial, especially when looking to establish a daily practice. These digital tools offer a convenient way to incorporate guided imagery and breathing exercises into your routine, balancing the mind and spirit. They can help maintain positivity and tranquility amid winter's often challenging atmosphere.

Workshops, whether in-person or online, also provide engaging opportunities to expand your winter wellness resources. These gatherings can range from cooking classes that focus on hearty and nourishing meals to yoga sessions that employ winter-friendly asanas. Participating in such activities fosters community and learning, helping you to integrate new habits and skills into your daily life.

Your physical space, too, plays a significant role in wellness. Creating a relaxation corner at home with cosy textiles, soft lighting, and personal mementoes can transform any nook into a sanctuary of comfort and introspection. Whether it's a plush blanket or a favourite scented candle, incorporating elements that bring you joy can turn your home into a haven against winter's chill.

For those invested in blending health with environmental consciousness, sustainable practices like eco-friendly ways to heat your home or cultivating an indoor winter garden can be both rewarding and enriching. These practices not only contribute to personal wellness but also foster a deeper connection with the world around you, all while respecting ecological values.

Lastly, don't underestimate the value of social connections as a resource for well-being. Whether it's virtual book clubs, online yoga sessions, or weekly chats with friends, engaging with others can significantly elevate your mood and sense of community. Sharing experiences, swapping stories, and simply being in the company of others—albeit virtually—can nurture the soul and make the darkest days seem a little brighter.

By integrating these resources into your winter routine, you create a tapestry of wellness that supports and sustains you. Each is a thread woven into your broader journey of embracing winter's challenges and opportunities. With an open heart and inspired mind, these resources empower you to thrive, not just survive, the winter months.

Further Reading and Inspiration

Embarking on a journey towards inner warmth and resilience during the winter months often intertwines with an unquenchable thirst for knowledge and inspiration. While this book provides a comprehensive guide, there's always more to explore beyond its pages. Immersing yourself in the wisdom and experiences of others can light the way as you cultivate well-being in the heart of winter's chill. This section highlights a selection of books, articles, and thought leaders whose work may further inspire and guide you.

The journey into personal growth and self-care is deeply enriched by the philosophy of embracing each season with gratitude and mindfulness. Works by authors such as John O'Donohue and David Whyte provide a poetic exploration of connecting with nature and finding beauty in the colder months. O'Donohue's insights into Celtic spirituality remind us to cherish the silent and introspective beauty of this season, offering solace and inspiration to those attuned to nature's cycles.

Reading is only one facet of exploration, though. Multisensory engagement can deepen your appreciation and understanding of winter's gifts. Podcasts focused on holistic living, like those led by thought leaders in mindfulness and well-being, offer invaluable audio companions on crisp winter walks. Listening to stories and insights from varied voices across the wellness spectrum can provide new perspectives and encourage active reflection about your own journey.

Seeking inspiration from non-traditional sources is equally enriching. The influence of traditional practices such as Ayurveda and Traditional Chinese Medicine (TCM) can lead you down a path of discovery. Books and resources that delve into these ancient practices provide intuitive insights into aligning your lifestyle with the rhythm of the seasons. Through understanding these systems, you can glean practices that resonate with your personal needs, particularly in how they address maintaining warmth and balance during winter.

An exploration of self-care and well-being in winter would not be complete without delving into the positive psychology movement. Esteemed authors and researchers in this field have offered a wealth of understanding about resilience and happiness that complements seasonal mindfulness practices. Consider the work of scholars such as Martin Seligman and Barbara Fredrickson, whose research highlights the profound effect of cultivating positivity and emotional resilience. Their findings can be particularly potent when applied during the darker, shorter days of winter.

The web of inspiration is wide, with the world of online communities offering another avenue for exploration. Websites and blogs dedicated to seasonal living and wellness provide not only practical advice but also a connective thread to like-minded individuals navigating similar desires to find harmony in winter. Online forums, where members share personal stories and tips on coping with winter's challenges, can foster a sense of community and shared experience.

In the spirit of creativity, don't overlook the power of art and creative expression to inspire and transform your winter experience. Reading books about art therapy or participating in creative workshops—whether they be about painting, crafting, or writing—can offer therapeutic pathways to process and express your winter reflections. Authors like Julia Cameron, known for her work on creativity as a spiritual practice, advocate for unlocking creativity as a means to deepen one's connection with oneself and the surrounding environment.

Delving into the works of scientists and wellness experts who focus on circadian rhythms can provide practical insights into optimising your health during winter. Books that explore the science of sleep and the influence of light on human biology are pivotal for understanding how to align your daily habits with your natural rhythms. Let the work of experts like Dr. Matthew Walker inspire you to cultivate habits that support restorative sleep and overall vitality during the colder months.

Every voyage towards self-awareness and inner warmth benefits from the companions met along the way and the inspirations drawn from them. The authors, researchers, and community leaders of these further readings serve as lanterns, guiding you with their informed insights and creative expressions. By engaging with their work, you not only expand your horizons but also enrich your personal journey towards embracing the transformative power of winter.

Remember, inspiration is not only found in words and theories but also in everyday practices, artistic expressions, and the shared wisdom of those who walk a parallel path. Whether you're listening to a podcast under a warm duvet, stepping out for a reflective afternoon wander with a new perspective, or diving into literature that speaks to your soul, each element weaves into the fabric of your winter resilience. Continue to seek it out and savour its impact, letting it kindle warmth within your heart long after the snow has melted.

www.ingramcontent.com/pod-product-compliance
Lightning Source LLC
Chambersburg PA
CBHW020422290526
45785CB00002B/684